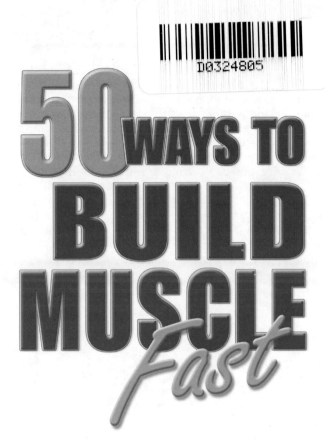

50 WAYS TO BUILD MUSCLE Fast

DAVE TUTTLE

AVERY PUBLISHING GROUP

Garden City Park • New York

The information and advice contained in this book are based upon the research and the personal and professional experiences of the author. They are not intended as a substitute for consulting with a health care profession-al. The publisher and author are not responsible for any adverse effects or consequences resulting from the use of any of the suggestions, preparations, or procedures discussed in this book. All matters pertaining to your physical health should be supervised by a health care professional. It is a sign of wis-dom, not cowardice, to seek a second or third opinion.

Cover designer: Oscar Maldonado
In-house editor: Karen Hay
Typesetter: Gary A. Rosenberg
Printer: Paragon Press, Honesdale, PA

Avery Publishing Group
120 Old Broadway
Garden City Park, NY 11040
1–800–548–5757
www.averypublishing.com

Publisher's Cataloging-in-Publication Data

Tuttle, Dave.
    50 ways to build muscle fast : the ultimate guide to building
bigger muscle / Dave Tuttle.
    —1st ed.
    p. cm.
    Fifty ways to build muscle fast
    Includes index.
    ISBN: 0-89529-951-8

    1. Bodybuilding. 2. Weight training.
3. Physical fitness—Nutritional aspects.
I. Title. II. Title: Fifty ways to build muscle fast

GV546.5 T88 1999   646.75
QBI99-1465

Contents

Acknowledgments

Many people have made contributions to this book through their thoughtful suggestions and technical assistance. I would first like to thank the experts in the field who generously gave their time so that you could benefit from their expertise. In alphabetical order, they are Anthony Almada, Dr. Mauro Di Pasquale, Kurt Elder, Marcus Elliot, M.D., Dr. William Kraemer, Dr. Pete Lemon, Karl List, Ray Sahelian M.D., Tomas Welbourne, Ph.D., and Dr. Richard Winett.

I would also like to thank my family and friends, who gave me the encouragement and support needed to make this book a reality.

Preface

Muscle. It's something that we all want, and the more the better. If you bought this book, then you agree that building muscle is an important part of your fitness program. Whether you seek additional strength to excel in your sport or just want to look good, you recognize that a muscular physique can bring many physical and psychological advantages, from increased lifting potential to greater confidence. You have seen how other athletes have achieved their goals, and you know that you can do it, too. This book will help you get where you want to go.

I have been a health and fitness writer for a decade, and I have trained with weights since the sixth grade. It's been quite a journey, and I have gathered a great deal of knowledge along the way. Through years of research, interviews with countless athletes, and my own high-intensity training, I have seen what works and what doesn't. Were there a few mistakes along the way? You bet, but over time I devised an excellent system for building muscle mass that I am now offering you in this book. Rather than learning through trial and error, you can now read about the most effective ways to pack on mass through the integrated approach discussed in these pages.

By incorporating these fifty ways to build muscle into your life, you will take your weight training to a new dimension. You will discover your true potential to build muscle in a healthy way that you can enjoy for years to come. You will gain mental and physical strength that will help you as you travel through life, and develop a physique that will increase the admiration of your peers. I wish you the best of luck on your journey.

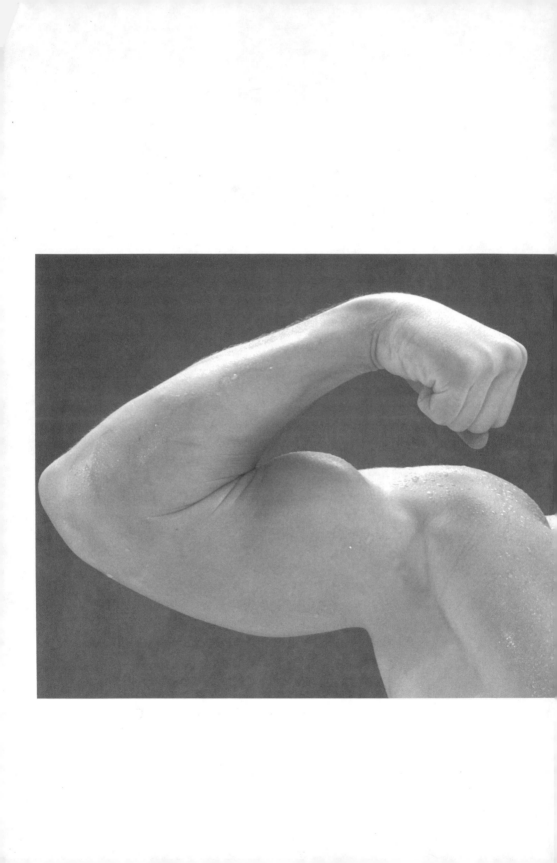

Introduction

YOU CAN DO IT!

Muscle mass is admired in our society. Most people look up to athletes who take the time to develop their bodies. People admire the hard work that goes into developing a muscular physique, even if they choose to focus on other activities themselves. They know the dedication and commitment that goes into a rigorous program of athletic training, and they respect the accomplishments of professional athletes. It has been this way for years, and it will continue to be for many more.

Congratulations on your decision to build more muscle! You will find that a muscular physique has a wide variety of benefits. Of course, increased muscle mass will improve your physical strength and give your body a more athletic shape. Yet, there is so much more. Achieving your muscular goals will help you in all aspects of your life. Once you meet this challenge, you will know that you can reach other life goals when you approach them with sufficient drive and intensity. However, none of this can happen if you just cross your fingers and wish for it.

You will find that there is a lot more to building muscle than lifting weights properly. While good form is essential to injury-free gains, it is just a small part of the big picture. There are many different variables involved in muscular development, and you will achieve your goals quickly when you incorporate all of them into your muscle-building program. I will highlight fifty of these variables in *50 Ways to Build Muscle Fast.*

Twenty-three of these variables relate to your training regimen. They include ways to structure your workout program for optimal effectiveness, plus techniques for getting the most out of every repetition and set. The next thirteen variables include recommendations for diet and supplementation. Most people have heard the adage that "you are what you eat," but they may not have made that connection with developing muscle mass. By the time you finish this book, you will recognize the full contribution that nutrition makes to muscle size. Another fourteen variables involve methods for integrating your workout into your overall lifestyle. While some people feel that the only time they affect their muscle growth is at the gym, you will find that you influence your growth potential twenty-four hours a day through your actions. We will look at everything from recuperation and overtraining to mental approaches for maximizing growth.

The human body is capable of amazing feats. While there are differences between individuals, most people are capable of reaching a level of muscular development that will set them apart from the crowd. Yet, some people will never achieve a superior physique because of their self-imposed limitations. In order to reach your maximum level of muscle mass, you have to leave these limiting factors behind you.

The power to transform your physique lies within you. Only through a full channeling of your mental and physical resources can you realize your dream of a totally muscular body. This book explains many different ways to achieve this goal. But above all, you must truly believe in yourself and your capabilities.

Focus on the potential you have within you, and pat yourself on the back when you make progress in your training. Establish your plan of attack and charge forward with confidence and determination. You know you want to build a powerful, muscular physique. Now make it happen. You can do it!

PART ONE

TRAINING TECHNIQUES

INTRODUCTION

You have undoubtedly heard that you need to train hard in order to build muscle. This is certainly true, but it is only part of the answer. Brute force and animal intensity are valuable assets in muscular development, but they are not the sum total of training technique. There is far more involved.

Part One discusses twenty-three different ways that you can pack on size at the gym. Some of these you may have heard about, but others have only recently been verified through scientific research. You will discover that there are many distinct methods for stimulating muscle growth, ranging from strategies that increase intensity to ways you can enhance the overall design of your workouts. You should incorporate as many of these training techniques as possible into your exercise program. The recommendations can build upon each other, creating mental and physical synergies that will allow you to achieve the greatest improvements in your physique. When your energies are focused in the same direction, you will find that you make the quickest gains as well.

This section of the book shows how you can personalize your training regimen to meet your own particular needs and constraints. It also gives you tips on how to pack the most punch into your exercise program without pushing yourself into the overtraining syndrome. However, keep in mind that what you do outside of the gym also impacts your progress. We will look at the contributions of diet, supplementation and lifestyle to your muscle growth later in this book. For now, let's explore how you can get the greatest benefit from your workouts.

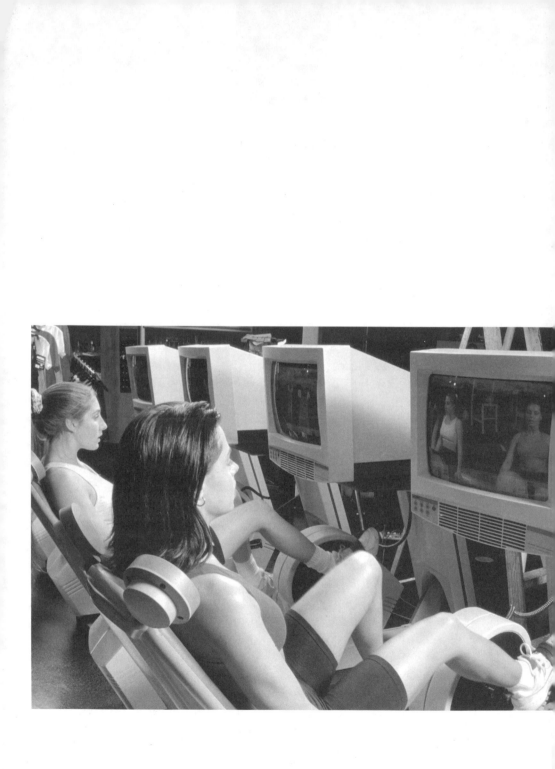

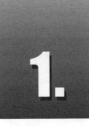

WARM UP
BEFORE YOU WORK OUT

A warm-up is an essential part of your exercise program. The increases in body temperature, heart rate, and other metabolic processes improve the speed of your nerve impulses. You should do a general body warm-up, a bodypart-specific warm-up, and an exercise-specific warm-up. All three types of warm-ups have their own distinct roles and benefits.

A warm-up helps you to get maximum results from your workout. Many people are in such a rush to begin their exercise routine that they either "forget" to warm-up or make excuses that it doesn't really matter. Nothing could be further from the truth. The warm-up provides the body with a necessary period of adjustment from the resting state to the active exercising state. Done properly, it can improve your performance while reducing the chances of injury.

There are many benefits to warming up. The temperature of the body increases, which improves the flow of blood through the muscles to be exercised. There is also an increase in the heart rate, which helps prepare the cardiovascular system for the work to come. Warm-ups improve the speed at which nerve impulses travel through the body, improving the efficiency of body movement. This allows the muscles to contract and relax with greater speed. A warm-up also increases the rate of certain metabolic processes and facilitates the release of oxygen from the blood.

All of these physiological changes enhance the work capacity of the body. The ability of the muscles and connective tissues to stretch and extend themselves improves, while the viscosity (or resistance to movement) within them decreases. Simply put, warming up readies your body for intense work while it gears up your mind to charge into the task at hand.

There are three types of warm-up: the general body warm-up, the bodypart-specific warm-up, and the exercise-specific warm-up. Each has a different role, and all are necessary for you to be fully prepared for your workout.

The general body warm-up should be the first thing you do at the beginning of a training session. This five- to ten-minute period of light exercise prepares the body for maximum performance and gives your mind the time it needs to focus on the coming workout, increasing your total efficiency and intensity.

The activity chosen, whether it be stationary biking, speed walking, rowing, stair climbing or the like, should be sufficient to raise the heartbeat and breathing rates and cause a bit of perspiration to form. It should not be so intense, however, that it becomes part of your regular workout. Some athletes do 100 percent intensity on their "warm-ups," figuring that anything less is not worth doing. This misses the entire point of warming up. You wouldn't think of driving your car on a cold morning without warming it up a bit. So why not give your body (the machine that you live in) the same benefit you give your automobile?

It is also necessary to warm up each bodypart before beginning high-intensity exercise. The bodypart-specific warm-up helps increase the flexibility of the muscle by allowing it to go through its full range of motion at an easy pace before beginning exercise at full-throttle. This movement increases the mobility of the joints and fine-tunes the muscle fibers for action, reducing the potential for injury. Bodypart-specific warm-ups help focus the mind on the specific muscle to be exercised, increasing the interaction between mind and muscle. This warm-up can also serve as the exercise-specific warm-up for the first exercise you do for a particular body-part.

The final type of warm-up is exercise-specific. This warm-up allows you to rehearse the actual movement and technique of an exercise before subjecting the muscle to a large amount of resistance. It also lets you make minor adjustments in posture that put you into proper position for execution of the exercise. This helps prepare the muscle for the heavier weights to come. The exercise-specific warm-up should be done using a weight that is 40 percent of your peak lifting weight for that day. On exercises such as squats that are performed with a great deal of weight, two warm-ups are often recommended. On the second warm-up, you should use a weight approximately halfway between the weight you used for the first warm-up and your peak weight, although you only have to do four to six repetitions on the second warm-up. (The goal here is to help prepare your muscles for the peak weight to come, not to tire them out.) This gradual increase in weight is called *pyramiding* and is a proven technique for maximum performance and injury prevention.

An exercise-specific warm-up should be done for every exercise you do. While some people feel that a muscle is entirely warmed up after a few sets, there are many different dimensions to a complete warm up. Each exercise can work the bodypart in a slightly different way. A quick warm-up set of eight to ten repetitions can be done in thirty to forty-five seconds. That's a small amount of time to invest in maximizing your growth potential.

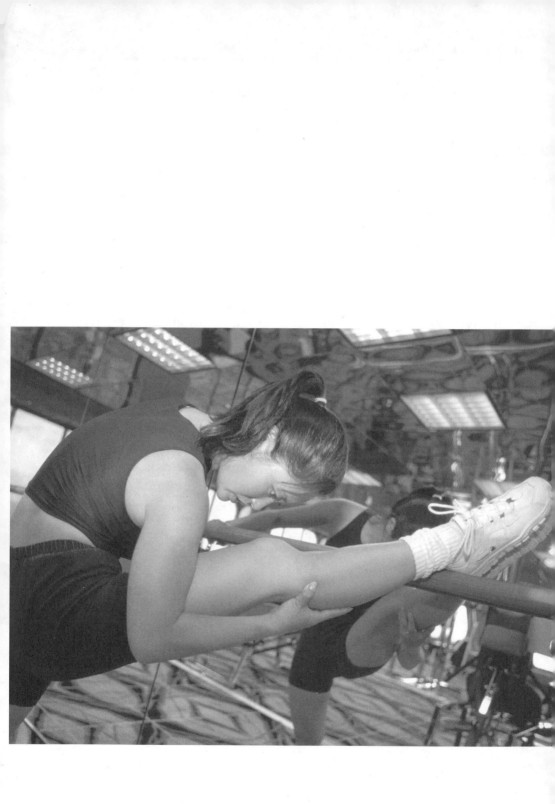

2.

STRETCH
YOUR MUSCLES

Stretching does more than increase flexibility. A slow, non-bouncing stretch, called a static stretch, can reduce immediate muscle soreness and increase a muscle's range of motion. As the muscle performs a more complete movement, larger forces are produced and greater muscular adaptations are stimulated. Be sure you don't strain the muscle, however. Stretch for ten to fifteen seconds before each set.

Stretching is a vital part of a complete workout. Besides increasing flexibility, it can enhance agility and coordination. This is particularly important in sports such as gymnastics and karate. Stretching can reduce stress through the relaxation of the muscle and help prevent injury to the joints and tendons. Properly done, it can also increase muscular strength.

A slow, non-bouncing stretch, called a static stretch, has been shown to reduce immediate muscle soreness. Everyone is familiar with the use of a stretch to relieve a muscle cramp. Research has now shown that static stretching decreases the electrical activity within skeletal muscle, which may explain why it is so effective for soreness. Care must be taken, however, to use the correct stretching technique. When performing a stretch, don't force the muscle to tense up by straining it. The whole point of stretching is to release tension, allowing the muscle fibers to elongate.

Visualize the muscle expanding as an elastic band would. Keep on lengthening the fibers slowly and without stress. If you feel a burning sensation or if the muscles start to quiver, you have gone too far. Ease off a bit. Of course, over time your muscles will adapt to these movements and become more flexible, allowing you to stretch them further without getting a pain sensation.

Done correctly, stretching can extend your muscles' range of motion. A muscle moves through only a portion of its total range during everyday life, so there is a significant reserve capacity. In weight training, however, you want to move the resistance through the fullest range of motion the muscle is capable of. Stretching allows you to move through a greater portion of this range, so the muscle fibers are able to contract over a greater distance than they would otherwise. Greater forces are therefore produced, stimulating additional muscular adaptations.

To be most effective in producing muscle growth, the stretch should be done after your body is warmed up. Stretch the body-part for ten to fifteen seconds immediately before each set. Pre-stretching a muscle activates certain nerve impulses in the muscle spindles and primes the muscle for the "stretch reflex," which (like any reflex action) causes a reaction to the initial movement. As the muscle moves through a greater range of motion, more muscle fibers are recruited. The end result is a stronger contraction and a greater amount of generated tension, which induces more muscle growth. Because the stretching is done during the rest period between sets, it does not prolong your workout. Stretching is therefore a wise investment of your time.

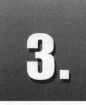

3.

VISUALIZE YOUR MUSCLES GROWING

Visualization is an important growth technique. By focusing your mind on a specific image, you can increase your motivation and achieve greater strength and size gains. The choice of visualization is yours, because only you know what will stimulate you the most. Try visualizing your workout the night before you go to the gym. During your set, enter a training trance. Visualize your muscles growing with each contraction. In time, the dream will become reality.

Visualization is an excellent way to maximize intensity. Through the use of mental imagery, you can achieve a level of concentration and focus that will push you harder than you ever thought possible. Everyone who excels in sports has a clear picture of where he or she wants to go. This picture should be as detailed as possible, so you can believe in the reality of it all.

Pick the visualization that is most effective for you. For instance, you could visualize that you are a machine. By the mechanical laws of nature you *will* achieve your goals! You are the ruler of your destiny, and you *choose* to dominate the weight with your unrestricted willpower. Or, you could use the imagery of the world around you. As you train, imagine your biceps becoming mountains of rock-hard muscle. Some track stars think of themselves as racehorses or greyhounds with powerful animal intensity. And most people, of course, want washboard abdominals, so envisioning that might help.

Concentrate on these images as you exercise each bodypart, developing different visualizations for particular muscles if this motivates you more. You could even alternate the images depending on your mood. These images don't have to "make sense" or be based on reality. If the visualization is effective, use it.

Think about these visualizations during the day. Most important of all, lock into them while you do your exercises. These positive images increase your intensity and help you to force out an extra repetition or two.

Some people find they increase their training intensity by visualizing a workout the night before they go to the gym. This should be done in a quiet, relaxing setting, such as a peaceful corner of your house or in bed before going to sleep. Going through the steps of a training session can help focus the mind on the task to come. It may even aid the subconscious in preparing for the next day's lifting.

To maximize the effectiveness of this method, remove all extraneous thoughts from your mind. This can be done in a variety of ways, ranging from meditation to more conventional relaxation techniques. Focus on one particular thought until it dominates your entire mind. This thought could be as simple as repeating the word "relax" over and over, or it could be a mantra like those used in Eastern meditation. Concentrating on your breathing may also help, especially if you count to ten while doing it. Another method is to alternate flexing and relaxing each bodypart, starting with your feet and continuing muscle by muscle until you reach your neck.

You'll probably find that thoughts pop into your head even when you don't want to think about them. Don't suppress these thoughts. You can't keep the genie in the bottle. Let all of them escape. Then your mind will be free to concentrate on the important task at hand: tomorrow's workout.

Visualize the exercises that you will do tomorrow and imagine yourself achieving the short-term goals you have set for that day. Picture the execution of the movements in your mind. Sure, the first few reps are easy, but you keep on going. Five, six, seven (they're getting harder now), but you dominate the weight. Now, visualize yourself pumping out that final repetition, fighting against a piece of iron that seems to get heavier by the instant. But you don't give in. No, you achieve the goal you have set for yourself. Mission accomplished. Now all you have to do is go to the gym and repeat the exercise.

With practice, you will be able to reach this level of focused concentration during each set. Withdraw from the world around you and enter a training trance where your entire consciousness centers on the performance of the exercise. During this trance, block out all of your other feelings and temporarily lose touch with reality. Lock onto the same thought patterns you focused on the night before. Breathe in the same slow, rhythmic way so that the trance "clicks in." (It may sound difficult, but it gets easier with time.) Become one with the movement. The resulting intensity will make a significant difference in your lifting performance.

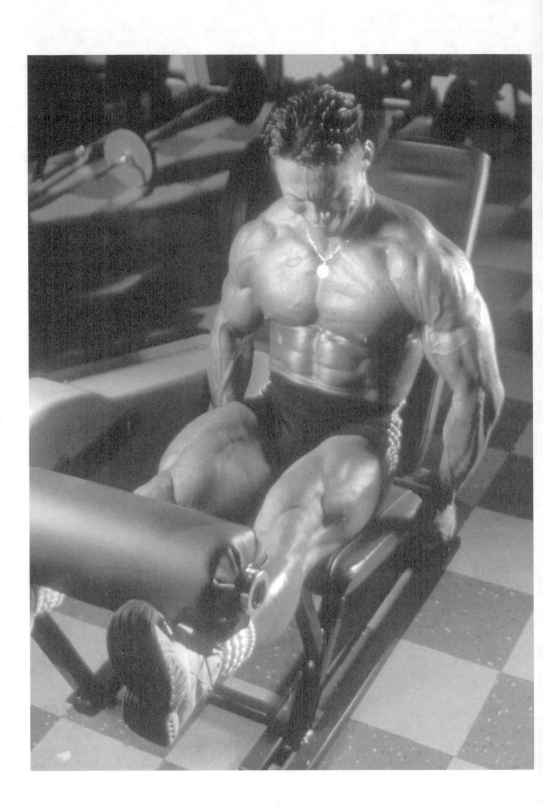

4.

DIVIDE YOUR MUSCLES INTO THREE OR FOUR GROUPS

While beginning athletes are able to make gains with a whole-body workout or a two-day split, more advanced athletes need to divide their bodyparts into three or four groups. These routines let you spend more time and effort on each muscle without creating excessively long workouts. This increases your intensity level and stimulates more muscle growth over time, provided that you train correctly. Be sure to include a rest day between bodypart cycles for recuperation.

Many athletes begin their weight training with a whole-body workout, in which all of the muscles are exercised on the same day. Later, they may divide their bodyparts into two separate routines. For example, the upper body would be trained on Day One and the lower body on Day Two. Both of these training regimens are productive for beginning athletes. Their bodies respond with a surge of growth as the muscles, unaccustomed to the rigors of progressive resistance training, pack on size. In fact, most athletes notice a considerable increase in strength and muscle mass during their first six months with the weights.

At some point, however, these gains begin to taper off. The body gets used to the demands placed upon it and stops growing at the same rate. In certain cases, the gains stop altogether. When this happens, you need to divide your muscles into three or four groups. With a three-day split you usually train three bodyparts per day. A four-day split allows you to train only two parts per day. The advantage of these training systems is that you can do more sets for each muscle without draining your body through excessively long workouts. This increase in training volume will stimulate additional growth over time.

Athletes who want to train a bodypart twice per week frequently use a three-day split. For example, you could train chest, shoulders, and triceps on Day One; quads/hamstrings, calves, and abdominals on Day Two; and back, biceps, and forearms on Day Three. This training system can be very effective. By giving each muscle two major doses of weight training each week, you stimulate your body to its maximum. As long as this greater volume does not push you into the overtraining syndrome, you will achieve significant muscle gains. Athletes who train for another sport at the same time, such as football players, often find that a three-day split performed once a week helps to increase their strength and size while still giving them enough time to train for their other event.

Four-day training cycles are becoming increasingly popular as a way to extend the time between bodypart workouts. With four-day splits, two bodyparts are usually trained each day. For example, you could train chest and shoulders on Day One; quadriceps/hamstrings and calves on Day Two; back and abdominals on Day Three; and arms on Day Four. The four-day system lets you perform even more sets per bodypart. It also allows more time for recuperation to occur. This may further increase your gains in muscle size and strength compared to the three-day system, provided, of course, that the muscles are trained at their maximum intensity during your workouts.

Although you may be tempted to get rid of your rest day to "make up" time, this is not a good idea. There are two types of fatigue: bodypart fatigue and systemic fatigue. A bodypart is fatigued when it has not fully recovered from your last workout. Soreness and reduced muscle strength are signs of bodypart fatigue. Systemic fatigue occurs when the entire body is stressed and overworked from the rigors of training. Your body can be systemically fatigued even if the individual bodypart you are scheduled to train is ready for another run with the weights. Since your body is still partially drained of its physical and mental energy, systemic fatigue keeps you from achieving your maximum intensity at the gym and should be avoided at all costs. Prolonged systemic fatigue can also result in illness. While it may seem counterintuitive at first glance, keeping a rest day in between training cycles can actually speed up your progress!

You may have heard that you must train a bodypart twice a week to make it grow. However, this is simply not true. Muscle growth is caused by an increase in the thickness of the muscle fibers. New muscle fibers can also be created in certain instances. These adaptations to weight training occur when the muscle is forced to respond to a resistance that it has not experienced before. Intensity is the key variable for muscle growth. You grow from that one set you did at a higher intensity level than ever before, not from volumes of submaximal training or too frequent workouts.

Many beginning fitness enthusiasts don't understand the dangers of overtraining, so they plunge into their workouts in a gung-ho manner that overwhelms their body's ability to recuperate and grow. This problem is discussed in greater detail in Part Three: Lifestyle. For now, remember that weight training is a peak-intensity sport, *not* an endurance sport.

The frequency of your training should be dictated by your recuperative abilities, not the day of the week. Your body doesn't know whether it's Tuesday or Friday. The body functions on much longer cycles, and athletes need to respect these fluctuations and work with them. You should never train a bodypart unless it has not been sore for at least a day. In time, you will actually be able to flex a muscle and determine whether it is sufficiently recuperated. If it doesn't feel that way, take another day off. If this means that you only train a bodypart three times in two weeks or even once a week, so be it.

Scientific research has shown that in healthy athletes the de-training process (where your muscles start to lose their strength through lack of use) doesn't start for two weeks, with significant losses taking up to a month. So don't worry about losing muscle if you don't train twice a week. In fact, for a committed athlete the chances of losing muscle through overtraining are greater if you *do* train twice a week. Train with total intensity, but train intelligently and in harmony with your body's abilities. In the long run, the muscle gains will be much greater.

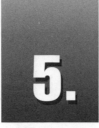

INCORPORATE TESTOSTERONE-RELEASING EXERCISES INTO YOUR WORKOUTS

Testosterone promotes muscle growth. Scientific studies have shown that two exercises, the squat and the powerlifting-style deadlift, produce a significantly greater release of testosterone than most other exercises. Always include these two exercises in your workout program. Pay particularly close attention to your technique on these movements.

Testosterone plays a major role in the growth and maintenance of muscle. This hormone stimulates increased muscle mass by helping to promote the buildup of muscle tissue (anabolic conditions). This is because the filaments within the muscle fiber that do the work of contraction are proteins (actin and myosin). Like all proteins, they contain nitrogen, which is derived from the protein foods we eat. Nitrogen can also be excreted from the body when tissue is broken down (catabolic conditions). By increasing the retention of nitrogen in the body, testosterone enhances protein synthesis and helps to ensure a positive nitrogen balance, which is when there is more nitrogen retention than excretion. It also decreases bodyfat levels and promotes the release of growth hormone.

Testosterone acts on the receptors on nerve cells as well, leading to changes in their structural protein content. This increases the ability of the muscle connected to these nerves to generate the forces required for muscle contraction. Most testosterone production in men occurs in the testes, although some takes place in the adrenal gland. Women also have testosterone, although usually only about 10 percent as much as men. It is produced in the adrenal gland. The pituitary gland secretes two hormones that control natural testosterone levels.

Scientists have known for many years that exercise stimulates the release of testosterone into the bloodstream. Recently, however, research has been done on individual exercises to determine whether they all produce the same hormone response. These studies by Kraemer, Fahey, Hakkinen, and others reveal that a significant release of testosterone is achieved during exercises that use large muscle groups, such as the powerlifting-style deadlift, power clean, and squat. These exercises stimulate testosterone production because a critical mass of the body's muscles is forced to contribute to the completion of the effort. This may not seem too surprising, as these exercises have long been considered mass-building power movements. However, studies by Guezennec and others show that the bench press does not produce a similar hormone release. This is because the body is stationary on a bench during that exercise, so the critical mass of body movement is not achieved.

"The larger muscle mass involved in the squat and deadlift increases the metabolic demands on the body to a critical level, which stimulates an endocrine response," says Dr. William Kraemer, Director of the Human Performance Laboratory at Ball State University. "The body recognizes that there is a need to repair itself after the exercise stress, so it produces testosterone and other hormones to carry out the task. Additional training adaptations are triggered as well, including up-regulation of various receptors and enhanced protein synthesis. Exercises that do not place such a metabolic demand on the body do not produce the same series of events." The inevitable conclusion: you should incorporate these testosterone-releasing exercises into your workout program for legs and back.

When the squat is properly performed, it can be a very anabolic exercise. Yet squats are frequently done with less than ideal technique, resulting in submaximal gains. The most frequent error is to place unnecessary strain on the lower back by leaning forward during the movement. When you descend into the squat position, your back should be perpendicular to the floor. While some forward motion is inevitable, this can be minimized when you place a 2 x 4 board or a five- to twenty-five-pound plate beneath the heels of your feet. Experiment to see which elevation works best for you.

Once you are in the squat position, think of yourself as a rocket. Thrust your body upward and not forward. Push up from the heels of your feet, which will help your balance. (This may seem like a small change, but it can make a big difference.) Also, look forward while you squat. Examine your technique in the mirror as you rise. Never look down, as this can cause you to lean forward, nor look up, which can result in a curving of the spine. Furthermore, when you lower your body into the squat position, make sure that your knees bend directly over your feet. Practice this without weights at first until you get it right. Knee problems are *not* inevitable with the squat. They result from improper technique. Minimize the strain on this essential joint by always making your feet "disappear" beneath your legs during the movement. This can be achieved with a close or wide stance, depending on how you pivot your legs at the hip.

The powerlifting-style deadlift is another potent testosterone releaser. In this exercise, the legs are bent when the weight is on the floor. The initial movement is with the legs, which begin the upward thrust of the body. This is very important. Sometimes novice athletes start this exercise with their backs, which is a great way to strain your lower back and injure yourself. After the legs begin the ascent, the upper body should follow suit until you are standing upright with your arms straight and the bar is in front of your legs.

Use a strap to grip the bar. This will allow you to focus all of your effort on maintaining perfect form during the upward thrust. The hands should be only as far apart as necessary to permit free clearance of the legs during the ascent. Some athletes alternate the grip of their hands, with one palm facing toward the body and the other facing away—this is said to improve balance. Others find this position awkward, and prefer to grip the bar with both palms facing the body. Use the position that you find most comfortable. This will allow you to focus all of your energies on the lift. Try to maintain the spine in a relatively straight position, without excessively curving it forward or backward. Such curvature places stress on the spinal column and can cause injury. This is particularly important at the top of the movement.

The inclusion of these two exercises in your workout will stimulate major muscle gains. The greatest testosterone release is achieved when you lift a weight that is 150 to 200 percent of your total body weight, although lower weights also produce a hormonal response. You should slowly work up to these ideal weights, however. Give your muscles plenty of time to adjust to the larger loads. In time, you will reach your goal without strain or injury. Patience is not only a virtue, it is a necessity for safe muscle growth.

In order to assure whole-body recuperation and to prepare yourself for this anabolic assault, take a break from training on the days before you do squats and deadlifts. If you can't take a day off because of your training schedule, at least try to separate the days you do squats and deadlifts in your routine as much as possible. This will spread these testosterone-releasing exercises throughout the week, permitting the most even distribution of this essential hormone over time. It will also give your legs more time for recovery, as both of these exercises utilize the thigh muscles to a great extent. This will stimulate the greatest amount of muscle growth and ensure that you reach your bodybuilding goals as soon as possible.

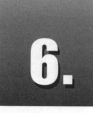

6.

GO FOR A FULL
RANGE OF MOTION

Exercising a muscle through its entire range of motion stimulates the greatest increases in size and strength. You should work the muscle from the fully stretched position to the fully contracted position on each repetition. While it is easier to do half-reps, they are far less effective for growth. Always use proper form, even if you have to temporarily lower the amount of weight that you use.

Every muscle has the ability to move through a certain range, or distance, at a specific joint angle. This full range of motion is often greater than the distance the muscle normally travels through. For example, relax your arms at your sides. They may appear to be fully extended, but contract your triceps completely. Your biceps get an additional stretch beyond their relaxed position. The biceps' full range of motion goes from this fully stretched position to the fully contracted position.

In order to get the greatest benefit from an exercise, each repetition should move through the muscle's full range of motion with perfect form. It's not as easy as it sounds. There is a big difference in the amount of weight you can lift at 80 percent of full range and at 100 percent. There is a tendency for the weight to "stick" where the mechanical lifting advantage is the smallest. Some people prefer to do 80 percent of their full range or even less so they can do more repetitions with heavier weights. Yet, while this technique may boost their egos, it keeps the muscles from growing as large as they could. In effect, these people are cheating themselves.

You should exercise the muscle's full range even if you have to temporarily lower the weight you lift to do the exercise with proper form. Of course, once you've perfected the technique and muscle growth occurs, you'll be able to lift the same weight that you did before (or even more) but now with excellent form. And you'll have bigger, stronger muscles to show for it!

The idea that half-reps stimulate growth is actually a half-truth. It is true that half-reps produce a certain degree of muscle growth. After all, muscular adaptations occur whenever force is applied against a resistance the muscle is unaccustomed to. However, you can only get so far with this technique. The greatest growth is obtained when the muscle passes through the entire distance that it is capable of moving through at a specific joint angle.

Proper form is a constant requirement for achieving your goals. Nothing will be gained by bouncing or "cheating" a weight up. You need to concentrate on your performance of the exercise, slowly moving through the entire range of motion with precision and care. Don't cheat yourself by stopping short of a full stretch and full contraction. Make each repetition count! This attention to detail will help ensure the greatest muscle stimulation.

7.

HOLD THE MOVEMENT AT THE POINT OF PEAK CONTRACTION

The point of peak contraction is where the muscle fibers are contracted, or shortened, to the greatest extent. When you reach this point, hold the position for a second before continuing the exercise. If you can't hold it there with the weight you are currently using, then lower the weight. Approach and depart from the point of peak contraction in a smooth, controlled movement.

As you move a weight during an exercise, some parts of the movement are more difficult than others. This is because gravity exerts a greater opposing force at certain times. For example, when you do a biceps curl, the beginning of the motion is relatively easy. As you continue to lift the weight, however, gravity makes the movement harder and harder until you reach the point of peak contraction. This is the point where all of the muscle fibers are contracted, or shortened, to the greatest extent.

In order to maximize your growth, you need to lift the weight to the point of peak contraction and then hold it there for a second.

This is easier said than done. Sometimes athletes stop short of a peak contraction because it is difficult or even impossible at the weight they are currently using. You now know the importance of moving through a muscle's full range of motion. Yet, reaching the point of peak contraction is not enough to achieve the largest possible mass. You must keep your muscle flexed at this point for a second to lock in your gains. If you can't hold the weight in this position, then lower the weight you use until you can perform the movement with perfect form. In time, your strength will increase and you will be able to lift the same weight you used to. Your muscles will respond to the extra stimulation with additional growth.

The way you approach and depart from the point of peak contraction is also important. Some athletes try to force the weight up in a jerky movement using momentum from other bodyparts. As soon as they reach the uppermost point of their movement, they let the weight drop back down to the starting position. This keeps the muscles from reaching their growth potential. You should contract your muscles with an explosive yet controlled movement that utilizes only the muscle or muscles you are training at that time. Momentum will not build mass. Although the total amount of weight you lift goes up, the amount of effort performed by the muscles you are targeting can actually drop. Relying on momentum denies your muscles the stimulation they want and need for growth.

As you approach the point of peak contraction, reduce the speed of your movement. You don't want to come to a screeching halt during an exercise any more than you would while driving your car. Gently "brake" on the muscle's motion until you come to a smooth stop. Hold this position for a second, then return to the starting position with a relatively slow movement that takes twice as long as the initial contraction movement. Never attempt to "catch" the weight after you have started your downward descent. This is a great way to injure yourself. When it comes to peak contractions, slow and steady wins the race.

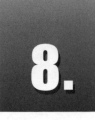

8.

REDUCE THE TIME BETWEEN SETS

By reducing the amount of time you rest between sets, you increase the intensity of your training program. You pack more muscle-building activity into a shorter period of time and stimulate more growth. The ideal rest period varies with the particular exercise, but as a general rule you should only rest one to two minutes between sets or until your heartbeat is back to normal, whichever is longer.

Another way to boost your training intensity is to reduce the amount of time you rest between sets. A more concentrated training program places larger demands on the muscle, which responds with greater growth over time. Although a certain amount of rest is necessary between sets to permit the short-term recovery of the muscle, too much of a break can hold you back. You need to walk the fine line between letting your muscles fully recharge for another set and giving them more time off than they really need.

The appropriate rest time between sets (or exercises for the same bodypart) varies with the muscle that is being trained. Larger muscles, such as the quadriceps, require more rest time than smaller muscles like the biceps and triceps. Also, compound exercises that involve several muscles, such as the squat and powerlifting-style deadlift, require longer rest periods than isolation exercises for a single muscle. This is a function of the demands you place on your body to lift the particular weights involved. The higher the exercise intensity, the more oxygen debt created and the more time you need to get your muscles back to a relatively recuperated state. There is also a build-up of lactic acid in and around the muscle during your set, which is largely neutralized during the rest period. This lactic acid is the cause of the "burning" sensation that forces you to stop contracting the muscle at the end of your set. A rest period also permits partial replenishment of the muscle's ATP supply (the fuel source for initial muscle movement) and other metabolic adjustments.

"Short rest periods have been shown to produce more testosterone and growth hormone secretion than longer rest periods when other factors are constant," notes Dr. William Kraemer, who is also co-author of the reference book *Designing Resistance Training Programs.* "Shorter rest periods also increase the number of capillaries inside your muscle fibers and boost the muscle's buffering capacity, which increases its ability to tolerate the build-up of lactic acid. These adaptations enhance endurance and contribute to muscle growth."

To achieve peak intensity, you should keep your rest periods as short as they can be while still providing time for appropriate recovery. A good rule of thumb is to rest one to two minutes between sets or until your heartbeat is back to normal, whichever is longer. (Your heart beats faster after you stop working out in order to get enough oxygen back into your system.) For most isolation exercises, a minute provides sufficient time to reduce the acidity in your muscles and to get them primed for more muscle action. Less than a minute is usually too little time for this recovery to take place. Anything much over a minute reduces your potential for peak intensity without giving you a compensating benefit in return. Compound movements require more recovery time due to their metabolic demands. One to two minutes is usually sufficient, however.

Remember that you are in the gym to grow. This is your prime directive, and you shouldn't let anything get in the way. You have undoubtedly seen athletes who spend three hours working out. You may wonder how anyone could do that many sets, but look closely the next time you see these people train. Chances are that they do a set, then rest five to ten minutes before doing another one. These prolonged workouts may be great for socializing, but they are not the best way to build muscle. The largest gains are obtained when you concentrate the greatest amount of training into the shortest period of time that is consistent with proper recovery.

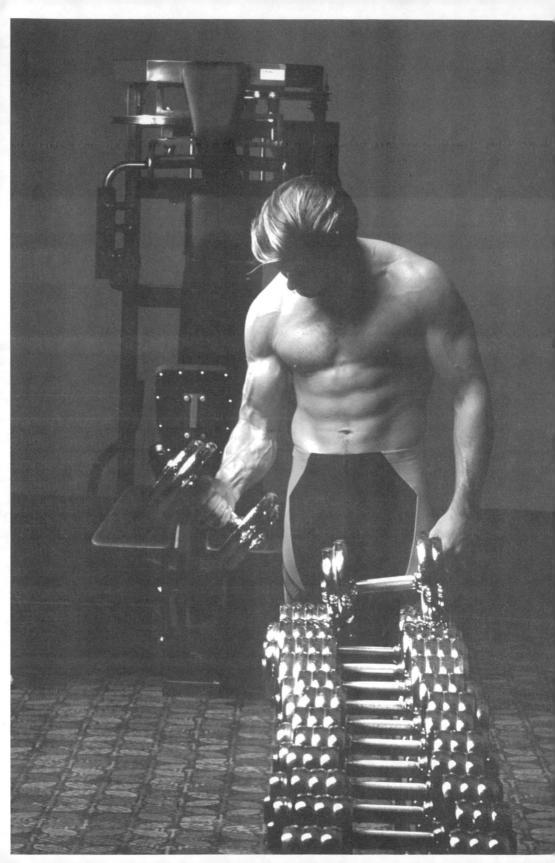

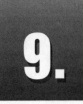

9.

FOCUS ON PROGRESSIVE RESISTANCE

Weight-training programs are based on the overload principle. When you increase the amount of weight you lift on a continuing basis, your muscle fibers adapt to these greater demands by gaining strength and size. If you are new to weightlifting, start with a weight light enough to do ten to twelve repetitions. After a couple of weeks, increase the weight by 10 percent and lower your repetition range to six to ten reps. Once you can do ten reps with that weight, increase the weight by 10 percent and slowly work up to ten reps again. Focus on progressive resistance. In time, you'll see major improvements in your physique.

Progressive-resistance exercise is a proven way to gain muscular strength and size. As you increase the amount of weight you lift over time, your muscles adapt to the ever-greater demands you place on them. When a muscle is exercised at an intensity that is close to its force-generating capacity, the muscle fibers increase in strength and eventually in mass. This mechanism is technically known as the overload principle. "Overload is the bottom line for muscle gains," says Dr. Richard Winett, editor of *Master Trainer* newsletter. "It provides the stimulus required for growth to occur. Every successful exercise protocol uses overload as its guiding principle."

When you begin weight training, you will have to determine the correct weights to use by trial and error. In general, you should select a weight that is 60 percent to 80 percent of your muscle's force-generating capacity. This is roughly equivalent to a weight you can lift for ten to twelve repetitions. This relatively high number of repetitions will allow you to adjust to the rigors of weight-lifting without placing an excessive strain on your untrained muscles. After a couple of weeks, your muscles will have adapted to your new workout program and you can safely increase the weights you use while reducing the number of repetitions.

As a general rule, the best repetition range for muscle growth is six to ten repetitions. Research has shown that this rep range produces the greatest size increases in the fast-twitch muscle fibers, which is the type of fiber predominantly recruited for weightlifting. Studies have shown fast-twitch growth with as little as four repetitions and as many as fifteen, but these numbers represent the edges of the bell-shaped curve. If you stick within the middle ranges of this curve, you'll get the most growth.

After you have completed your initial adjustment to weight training, you should pick a weight that will allow you to do an average of six repetitions on each set of an exercise. The next time you do that exercise, do at least one more repetition per set. This will increase your rep count to seven or maybe even eight. When you can do an average of ten repetitions on each set, increase the weight you lift by approximately 10 percent. Of course, this will reduce the number of repetitions you can do, but since the weight you are lifting has gone up, you are still achieving overload. Let's say, for example, that the number of reps you do drops to an average of six with your new weight. The next time you do that exercise, aim for an average of seven, then eight, nine, and ten. Once you are again up to an average of ten, increase the weight once more. This process can continue for many years.

Sometimes athletes do higher repetition ranges in an attempt to train their slow-twitch fibers, which is the type predominantly used for submaximal activities such as running. However, this technique is not really effective. First, slow-twitch fibers don't grow as much as the fast-twitch fibers. Second, these fibers only respond to a significant degree from rep ranges that are greater than twenty, usually much greater. How many thousands of repetitions does a runner do, for example? The best strategy for muscle growth is to develop your fast-twitch fibers through weightlifting and then do a limited amount of aerobics for your slow-twitch fibers. This will produce the greatest overall mass.

You should begin lifting your maximum weight just as soon as you are fully warmed up. Sometimes athletes do three or four warm-up sets before they reach their maximum weight. One or two of these sets, of course, are necessary to ensure that the muscle is completely warmed up and ready for action. Powerlifters who are warming up to do one-repetition maximal lifts will often need to do more than this. Yet for most other athletes, any more than two submaximal warm-up sets will needlessly tire out the muscle without providing any benefit in return.

Always do your sets to failure. Don't stop just because you reach the number of repetitions you originally had in mind. Push yourself to the maximum. If you were planning on doing eight repetitions and find that you can do ten, this means that it's time to increase the amount of weight you are training with. You need to keep on raising the amount of weight you lift with good form so your muscles are stimulated to grow in strength and size.

To achieve the greatest power for your exercises, raise the weight in a controlled yet explosive movement. These rapid concentric contractions should be done as swiftly as possible while still using proper exercise technique. Speed is never an excuse for sloppiness. Then, lower the weight relatively slowly to its original position, but never so slowly that you do a prolonged negative movement. This will produce the greatest gains in power with the least amount of muscle soreness.

Weightlifting is not an endurance sport. It is a peak-intensity sport based on the overload principle. Your muscles grow from the one set when you lift more than you ever did before, and not from the ten sets you did at a weight you have lifted for years. As was noted earlier, overtraining your muscles by doing excessive numbers of sets is not the way to achieve maximum muscle strength and size. You have to aim for peak intensity through progressive resistance, not muscular burnout. If you have trained a muscle so hard that it can no longer perform at its maximum, either switch to another bodypart or leave the gym. Once you find the right combination of training volume and frequency that allows you to achieve progressive resistance on a continuing basis, you will see major improvements in your progress.

10.

FOLLOW THE NATURAL PATH OF YOUR MUSCLES

Nature designed our muscles, bones, and tendons to work together as a unit. Muscles are able to generate the greatest force when they are trained on their ideal planes of motion, so you should always work your muscles along these planes. Exercising muscles at odd angles does not stimulate more growth or change the shape of your muscles. Athletes also risk injury when they resort to these unusual positions.

Muscles allow the body to stand upright and move in a coordinated fashion. Each muscle connects two bones, and the entire network of skeletal muscles and bones is called the "bony lever system." Muscles are connected to the outer coating of the bones by tendons, which are strong and densely constructed connective tissues that allow the force of muscular contraction to be transmitted from the muscle cells to the outer reaches of the bones. These muscles, bones, and tendons work together as a unit to allow a wide variety of physical movements.

The point at which the tendon connects to the relatively stable part of the skeleton is called the muscle's *origin*. The point where the tendon attaches to the bone that performs the movement is known as the *insertion*. The locations of these origins and insertions are permanent, and cannot be modified through training. Therefore, if a person has a genetically short biceps, this muscle trait will always remain. The biceps can increase in size through muscle growth, but it cannot grow outward by changing its connection points to the bones. This is one of the "givens" that we all have to live with.

Sometimes athletes are told that they can change the shape of their muscles by performing unusual movements. For example, you may have heard that rotating your ankles inward while doing a calf raise will work the outer part of your calf muscles. Unfortunately, this "technique" is erroneous. The tendons for the two calf muscles (gastrocnemius and soleus) are both attached to the back of the foot, not the sides. The function of the calf muscles is to raise the body to the tiptoe position, not to rotate the ankles inward and outward. (Other muscles are involved in these movements). Since the calves are not recruited for these rotations, they cannot be a factor in calf growth. However, when you perform a calf raise with these odd positions, you do bring into play a number of smaller muscles that are more easily strained. This increases the risk of injury without improving the growth potential of your calves one iota. This is a lose-lose situation that you should definitely avoid.

The chest, back, and shoulder muscles are able to operate on broader planes of motion. For instance, the main chest muscle (pectoralis major) can move the arm in a variety of directions because it has many points of origin along the breastbone. However, for most muscles there is only a single point of origin and insertion and, as a result, one ideal way to lift a weight. Muscles are able to generate the greatest force when they are trained on these ideal planes of motion, so you should always work your muscles along these planes. It is here that the mechanical advantage for lifting is the greatest and the muscles are most "comfortable" at performing their function.

Athletes usually recognize when they are training a muscle in a disadvantageous position. They frequently get warning signals from their muscles or tendons in the form of pain or unusual sensations informing them that their technique is off. Yet, athletes sometimes interpret these signals as a call to action. They recall the "no pain, no gain" credo and figure that if it hurts, it must be valuable for growth. Nothing could be further from the truth. Your body is trying to keep you from injuring yourself, so listen to the warnings it is giving you. Your muscles and your mind have to work together. When they do, you win with a new spurt of muscle growth.

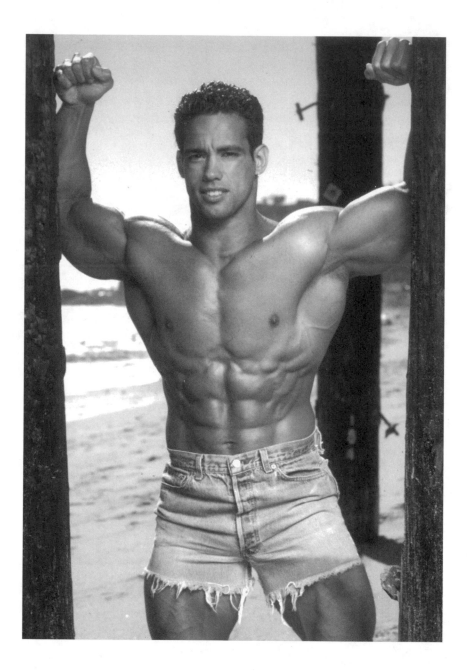

11.

INCORPORATE ISOMETRICS INTO YOUR WORKOUTS

Isometric exercise can boost your gains by providing another stimulus for muscle growth. After a set of progressive resistance exercise, maintain isometric tension for fifteen to twenty seconds without holding your breath. Strength gains from isometrics are specific to the joint angle trained, so try to mimic the action you did during your set as much as possible.

Isometrics is an effective but often-ignored way to gain strength. An isometric contraction occurs when a muscle contracts against an object that does not move. For example, when you force the palms of your hands together, you are performing an isometric contraction for your pectoral (chest) muscles. Isometrics provides an additional stimulus that the muscles can respond to over and above that provided by progressive resistance training. Research has shown that isometrics can produce strength gains and muscle growth when the isometric contractions are maximal and are performed on a regular basis.

Charles Atlas first promoted isometric exercise in his famous

Dynamic Tension course in the 1950s, which advocated isometrics as the sole means of gaining strength. By itself, however, isometrics is no match for weightlifting. Studies have since proven that when used alone, isometrics is far less effective than regular weight training for enhancing muscle strength. In fact, rumor has it that Charles Atlas gained his celebrated physique by occasionally pumping the iron.

Yet, when used in combination with progressive resistance training, isometrics can give you a supplemental means of developing strength. However, the strength gains from isometric exercise are joint-angle specific. This means that the increase in strength is found only within a range of plus or minus 20 percent of the joint angle at which the isometric exercise is performed. This specificity principle can be used to advantage when trying to increase strength at a sticking point, which is the joint position where a movement is most difficult to perform (that is, where the mechanical advantage for lifting is the smallest). Performing an isometric exercise at this joint angle will help you gain strength at this crucial point, improving your performance potential for the entire exercise. This technique is called functional isometrics.

Wrestlers find this isometric strength especially helpful, since many of their holds are isometric in nature. Bodybuilders benefit because flexing is also a form of isometrics. So try adding some isometrics to your routine. Immediately after your set, maintain isometric tension for fifteen to twenty seconds without holding your breath. For example, after you do dumbbell flyes for chest, you could press your hands against both sides of the bench you used for that exercise. Be sure to mimic the joint angle you used for the flyes as much as possible. When tension is applied to the already exhausted muscle, an additional growth stimulus is provided. It's kind of like doing forced reps, but without the weight.

Since most people take at least sixty seconds between their sets, this isometric movement basically occupies dead time and puts it to good use. It therefore makes the exercise a form of superset without moving between (and trying to save) two pieces of equipment. Also, once you get the feel of the isometric movement, you will be able to perform it in an inconspicuous manner that will not arouse attention. So add isometrics to your weight-training program. Your strength will increase faster than with weights alone. Greater muscle mass will be the welcome result.

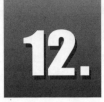

TRAIN WITH
A BUDDY

A training buddy can increase the intensity of your workouts. He or she can help you force out a few additional repetitions and motivate you to perform at your best. Picking the right partner is important. You need someone who arrives on time and is serious about his or her training. Once you find this person, try to make the relationship work. The mass gains that you both achieve will make it worthwhile.

Training with a buddy can recharge your workouts. While it is always important to be self-motivated, a buddy can reinforce your own drive and help you to achieve your goals. He or she can give you that extra push by creating a more positive training environment. When you both share the same muscle-building objectives, your personal energies can feed off one another's to create an even greater energy level. It's good to know that someone is there for you, especially when you are lifting heavy weights. Also, if your mind wanders or your intensity slackens, a buddy can provide support and encouragement.

A training partner can spot you when you need it. If you train by yourself, you are limited to the number of repetitions you can successfully complete without assistance. You may even need to stop short of the maximum number of reps due to safety factors. Athletes who perform barbell bench presses, for example, often have to hold back so they don't wind up with several hundred pounds of iron resting on their chests. A buddy can gently lift the weight while steadying the path of the barbell. He can also shout out motivational messages that will help you perform additional reps.

Make sure that your partner doesn't do too much of the work for you. He or she should lift up the bar or dumbbell just enough to let you complete the repetition. If he or she does more than this, he or she is actually robbing you of potential muscle gains. Your buddy is not psychic, however, any more than you are. Inform your partner when he or she spots you more than you need, and ask this person to do the same when it is your turn to spot. The combination of minimal spotting assistance and maximal motivational support will spur both of you on to greater muscle mass.

It's important to pick the right buddy, however. You need to find someone who is punctual and driven to succeed. Nothing can be more frustrating than waiting for a partner who is habitually late. Of course, everyone is tardy once in a while because of traffic jams or unexpected emergencies. However, if this lateness occurs regularly, then your partner may be holding you back. When you arrive at the gym, you should be psyched for your workout and raring to go. If your buddy is unwilling or unable to stick to the schedule you have agreed on, try to find another partner who is more focused on progress.

You also need a buddy who can motivate you to excel. This does not necessarily mean that your partner is stronger than you are. You could both be at the same strength level or your buddy could even be less advanced in his training. The important thing is that you work well together. If your partner is more interested in chatting about last Saturday's party or yesterday's sports scores, he or she may actually drain you of motivation. Although socializing is an important aspect of life, now is not the time for it. It's important to keep your intensity level high so you can blast past your limitations. Your buddy should help you do this. If this partner doesn't, find a new one.

At the same time, you shouldn't ditch a partner just because he or she is late once or is occasionally in a chatty mood. As with all relationships, you need to show a bit of flexibility. This person may not be perfect as a training buddy, but you are probably not pure perfection yourself. Look at the benefits you are receiving and compare them to the negatives. If you sense a need for improvement, talk it over with your buddy. He or she may not realize what he or she is doing, and may appreciate a kind word of advice. Look for ways that you can help each other gain the muscle you are both looking for. It may take a while to reach an acceptable arrangement, but the shirt-stretching mass you both achieve will be the welcome prize.

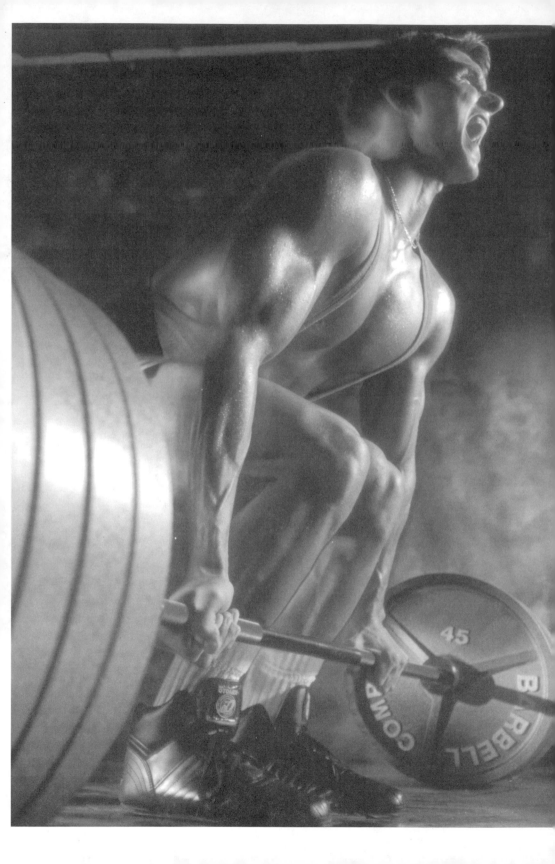

13.

BE INTENSE ABOUT YOUR WORKOUTS

You can't pack on size by going through the motions in a nonchalant manner. You have to be intense about your training. This intensity level is largely determined by your mindset. Focus on increasing your motivation, confidence level, and drive.

Sometimes you see people at the gym who go through their workouts in a lackadaisical way. They perform their exercises with minimal effort, occasionally chatting with friends during the actual movement. These people never seem to grow. Coincidence? Hardly. In order to build muscle you have to approach your workout with maximum intensity.

Many factors determine your intensity level, including your motivation, goal orientation, confidence level, and drive. Intensity is really independent of your strength, although some people confuse the two concepts. A novice athlete who lifts twenty-five-pound dumbbells, using every bit of determination he or she can muster, has a higher level of intensity than a larger or more developed athlete who lifts thirty-five-pound dumbbells with a nonchalant "what-me-worry" attitude. Won't the more "advanced" athlete be surprised when the novice's intensity level stimulates so much muscle growth that he starts lifting forty-five-pound dumbbells, bypassing the level of the other athlete!

The intensity you achieve is dependent on your mindset. Lifting a weight is a simple case of mind over matter, in which the mind sends neural impulses to the muscle ordering it to lift the weight. As a result, the amount of weight you can lift is frequently determined by the amount that you think you can lift. This is the major reason why athletes of the same height, age, and body type can lift widely varying amounts of weight. To a significant degree, the boundaries of individual accomplishment are set by the person's self-esteem.

You need to believe in yourself and your ability to achieve what you set out to do. Only when you are confident of your direction in life will you be able to rise from the mass of athletes and soar to your true potential. It is not enough to believe that you *may* get stronger. You have to believe that you *will* get stronger, just as the sun rises every day. Rather than letting yourself fall victim to negative thoughts, block them out and fill yourself with positive mental programming. Don't take *no* for an answer!

You can set a positive course for your training and by-and-large stick to it. The self-image each of us has determines what we can and cannot do. If this self-image is expanded, a whole new range of opportunities opens up. The choices are personal, but the methodology is the same for everyone. Believe in yourself and most of the battle is won. Once this is accepted, the excuses have to stop. The will to excel comes from within. High levels of intensity are possible if the mind wants them badly enough. Mental power, properly focused, will allow you to reach your full potential in sports.

14.

SET REALISTIC GOALS

Goals give you specific targets to shoot for. They build confidence and charge up your mind with energy and will. Set short-, medium-, and long-range goals for your muscle development. Short-term goals should be easily accomplished so you can savor victory on a regular basis. Your medium- and long-range goals will give you direction and staying power, helping you to ride out the bad times. All are essential to boosting size and strength.

Successful athletes know the importance of goalsetting. Without the focus that a goal provides, the energy of the mind is scattered like sand in the wind. Goals help you persevere through the tough times because your efforts are part of a larger picture. Your temporary sacrifices are then worth it, because each day brings you closer to the achievement of your goal. This helps to keep you from getting discouraged when you hit sticking points in your training.

Goalsetting can make a major difference in your muscular development. A nebulous desire is not sufficiently detailed to charge the mind with energy and willpower. You need a specific target to shoot for, something you can clearly see in your mind.

It is important to set short-, medium-, and long-range goals for your exercise program. It's fine to have a long-term goal of going to the Olympics, but if you're just starting out in a sport the achievement of that goal may be so far in the future that it winds up depressing you instead of providing inspiration. While it's true that a journey of a thousand miles begins with the first step, you need to focus on the fulfillment of each of those steps rather than spending all your time dreaming about the thrill of victory as they put that gold medal around your neck. Always keep that long-range goal in the back of your mind, however, so you can tap into it when the need arises.

Your short- and medium-range goals need to be realistic enough to help you sustain your efforts on a day-to-day basis. Don't bite off more than you can chew. Choose a goal that you have an excellent chance of achieving, say, doing one more repetition on your barbell curls. This goal is modest in the grand scheme of things, but it should be well within your grasp. Go for it and achieve it! Savor the satisfaction that comes from reaching your goal, but don't gloat on your newfound strength. Set another goal for your next workout. Aim for another repetition on each set or an increase of five to ten pounds. This will build upon your previous successes and help you reach a medium-range goal, such as winning a local competition or achieving a certain bodyweight.

If your goals are realistic, and you approach the task with determination and drive, while giving your body sound nutrition, you will reach the goals you have set. Don't let anything get in your way! Approach this challenge as you would any other that you confront in your life. And remember to pat yourself on the back when you accomplish a short- or medium-range goal. You may not have reached your ultimate goal yet, but let yourself feel the satisfaction and pride that comes with goal achievement. These positive feelings, and the self-confidence that comes along with them, will speed you on your way to the long-term goal you have set.

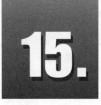

VARY YOUR WORKOUTS

Variety is the spice of life. Anything done to excess is boring, and weight training is no different. If your gains have stopped or even slowed down, you can get back on the right track by adding variety to your exercise program. There are many excellent ways to vary your workouts. Variation will unlock the power of your mind and body. This will increase the commitment to your training program.

One of the secrets to maintaining enthusiasm in weight training is variation. It would get boring to eat the same thing for dinner every night, and an exercise routine is no different. The best way to create excitement and stimulation for your workout is to constantly vary the elements of your training program. This fresh approach will increase your intensity level dramatically.

If you've been using the same routine for an extended period of time, your body may have gotten used to it. "The body can't stand redundancy," notes Dr. William Kraemer. "If you do the same thing all of the time, your body's adaptation mechanisms tend to shut down. You have to continually provide the muscles with new and different stimuli to achieve muscle growth." If your strength or size gains have stopped or if you're bored with the same old workout, it's time to try something new. Variation will bring back the spark to your training and get you on the right track again.

"You need to maintain an open mind," says exercise physiologist Karl List. "Don't get attached to any one training model. Try different things so you can see what works for your own body." There are many different ways to vary your workout. The number or type of exercises can be changed. Some days you could do three exercises for a bodypart, and on other days two or four. This could mean raising or lowering the number of sets you do for each exercise (so the total number of sets remains constant), or you could have high-volume and low-volume days. You could also change the order of the exercises and/or the order in which you train your bodyparts. Modifying the weights and number of repetitions per set is another alternative.

You could also switch the exercises you do. These variations in your routine should spice up your training, providing a new basis for growth. New exercises often work the muscle in a slightly different manner, which can stimulate the muscle fibers in distinct ways. Another option is to alternate the type of exercises, doing only compound movements with free weights for a while and then switching to machines or isolation movements. Or you could try concentrating on pressing exercises one day and cable movements the next.

Experiment with your routine to see which variations work best for you. There is no reason to stick with a group of exercises just because you got good results. Something else may be even more effective. If not, go back to your first workout or try yet another variation. Variety is the key to unlocking the power of your mind and body, and there are so many possible variations that there is no reason to be bored with your routine. Seek out new options. Explore the possibilities. You'll grow more and have more fun to boot.

16.

PERIODIZE YOUR
TRAINING PROGRAM

Periodization is a systematic way to program variation into your workouts. Instead of training at peak intensity all of the time, you structure your intensity levels in a way that permits long-term recuperation and growth. Start by taking a short break from training. Then ease into your periodization by lowering your intensity by 30 percent. For the next eight to ten weeks, slowly increase the weights you use and the number of repetitions you do. After a two- to three-week phase of lower intensity, begin a new periodization cycle. In the long run, you'll make bigger gains.

A well-designed periodization program is essential for optimal growth. By working in sync with your body's growth patterns and limitations, you can ensure that the maximum growth stimulation is provided at the right times and in the right amounts. Excessive training is avoided, along with the frustration and disappointment that often comes with it. An organized arrangement of intensity and volume fluctuations provides the ever-increasing stimulation required for muscle growth without pushing your body into over-training. Instead of playing it safe by constantly applying a sub-maximal level of force, you can give your all at the gym for certain periods without fear of overtraining. During these high-intensity weeks, you can force your muscles into a growth response by lifting more weight and/or doing more repetitions than you have done previously. Then you give your muscles some time to consolidate their gains and build a foundation for future growth. In this way, programmed change will lead to consistent size gains.

Periodization is frequently done by powerlifters, who start out with relatively light weights and large numbers of repetitions at the beginning of their training programs and then gradually increase the weights while reducing the repetitions per set as the day of the competition gets closer. Competitive athletes in other sports schedule their periodizations to coincide with their meets as well, timing everything so they reach the event in peak condition. Athletes who don't compete can use shorter periodizations year round.

Periodization programs have several different phases. Athletes often begin by taking a short break from training, usually a week or two. This gives the body time to recharge before beginning this high-intensity program. Be realistic about the break you need. Don't jump back into your training regimen before you have fully recovered from your previous routine. At the same time, don't use it as an excuse to "kick back" once your muscles are replenished and ready for action. The amount of time should be just right, allowing you to be mentally and physically refreshed and eager to return to the gym.

The next step is to ease back into your training regimen. Initially, start with weights that are 30 percent less than the weights you were lifting before your time off. Concentrate on your exercise technique, making sure that each repetition is done perfectly. Feel the movement of the muscle. For now, do only as many reps as you did with the higher weight you were using before your time off, even though you will not reach total failure. Resist the temptation to go all out with this lighter weight, which would just mean doing a higher rep range. You should be warming up your body for greater intensity later on. Just as you would let your car warm up a bit before you floor the accelerator, give your body a chance to ease into your new workout program.

Now, every time you train, slowly add more weight and intensity while staying within a rep range of six to ten. (Some sports will use lower rep ranges.) Keep a training log so you can be scientific about this. In time, you will surpass your former sticking point. When your gains start to stagnate again, begin another periodization.

The precise length of your periodizations will vary depending on your particular sport and competition schedule, but the usual length is eight to ten weeks. After this period, drop the intensity level at least 30 percent for two to three weeks. If you still feel overtrained after this two to three week break, take an entire week off from the gym. You need a break. Then begin your next periodization.

There aren't many athletes who systematically practice periodization. Yet many people wind up periodizing involuntarily by their own actions. Sometimes weightlifters are so compulsive about their training that they work out even when their bodies can't cooperate due to stress or other factors. If this happens too frequently, you may literally become sick. Then what happens? You take a week or two off, go back to the gym and find that the weights you can lift are down by about 30 percent. Now you slowly work your way back up to where you were before, in time surpassing your previous record. Sound familiar? Getting sick is an example of involuntary periodization, and unfortunately this is the only type of periodization that many athletes know. Yet, why wait until your body protests through illness to practice this training strategy? Get ahead of the game by adding periodization to your workout program.

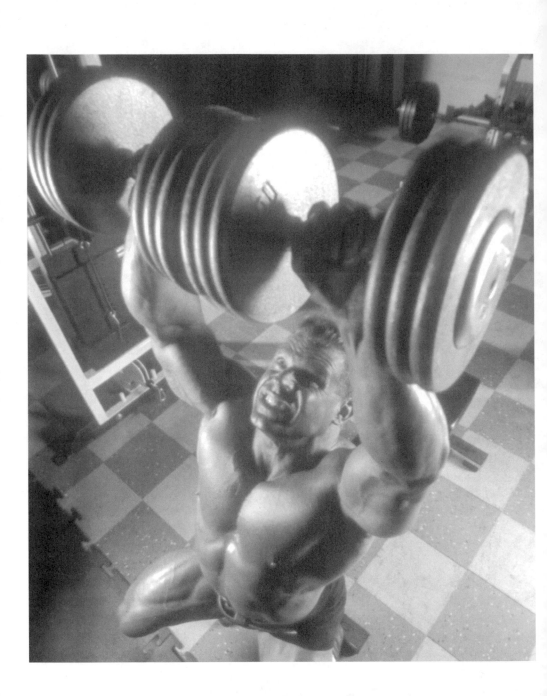

17.

USE SUPERSETS AND COMPOUND SETS

Performing two sets together without a rest period can also stimulate growth. A superset works the muscles on both sides of a joint, such as the biceps and triceps. One set for each bodypart is done without a break in between. A compound set includes two exercises for the same bodypart. Both techniques are effective as long as your workout volume doesn't push you into the overtraining syndrome.

Supersets and compound sets are tried-and-true ways to boost intensity. By eliminating the rest period between sets, you increase the volume of training per unit of time. This greater intensity will enhance your growth prospects, provided that you don't overtax your body and wind up overtraining yourself.

Supersets work the muscles on both sides of a joint. They take advantage of the "agonist-antagonist" relationship between specific pairs of muscles. For example, when you do a biceps curl, your triceps stretch out. Likewise, when the triceps shorten, the muscle fibers in the biceps elongate. If they didn't, your muscles would be locked in conflicting positions and you wouldn't be able to move. Scientists describe this complementary association as agonist-antagonist. When a muscle on one side of a joint is exercised, the muscle on the opposite side is also exercised to some extent. This beneficial relationship can make supersets very effective.

Moving immediately from an exercise for an agonist to another for its antagonist heightens the intensity level for *both* muscles. It may also provide needed variation to your workout program, since most athletes train biceps/triceps, chest/back, and quadriceps/hamstrings on different days. Training these agonist/antagonist muscle pairs at the same time may give your muscles the surge of intensity they have been "longing for." Supersetting will also permit the greatest amount of recuperation time within a bodypart rotation. Arms are trained on a single day instead of getting half workouts on two days. These alternating patterns of intense exercise and recuperation permit greater recovery from the stresses of training and promote more muscle growth.

Just be sure to use a spotter when you train two large bodyparts on the same day. You may find that you are able to lift less weight toward the end of your workout than you did when you trained each bodypart separately. Don't be alarmed about this apparent reduction in strength, however. The important thing is the total intensity achieved and the amount of long-term growth that you are stimulating. In order to promote the most even muscle development, alternate the bodypart that you begin with. For example, start your arm workout with biceps during your first training session and switch to triceps for your next workouts.

Compound sets are two exercises for the same bodypart that are performed without a rest in between. This technique can really pump up your muscles by giving them a high level of exercise intensity in a short period of time. Remember how many repetitions you did at a particular weight load for each exercise when you did them separately, then perform both sets without a break doing at least this many repetitions for each exercise while using the same amount of weight. Compound sets can trigger substantial new growth when done appropriately.

A compound set can also be used to overcome differences in the rate that muscles develop. In a perfect world, all muscles would grow at the same pace. Unfortunately, most athletes have some muscles that respond more quickly to training stimuli than others. One way to eliminate these lagging bodyparts is to perform compound sets *only* for these muscles. This will provide relatively greater intensity to your slower-growing bodyparts and bring them up to the high standard of muscular development of the rest of your physique over time.

To ensure that supersets and compound sets do not overburden your body, be sure to count each of the exercises you do as one set. That way, there will not be an increase in the total volume of training, merely an increase in intensity due to the reduction in time between sets. Once your body has adjusted to this new stimulus, you can experiment with higher training volumes by considering each superset or compound set as a single set in your workout program. However, even then you shouldn't do more than two supersets or compound sets per bodypart. These techniques are most effective when they are the exception instead of the rule.

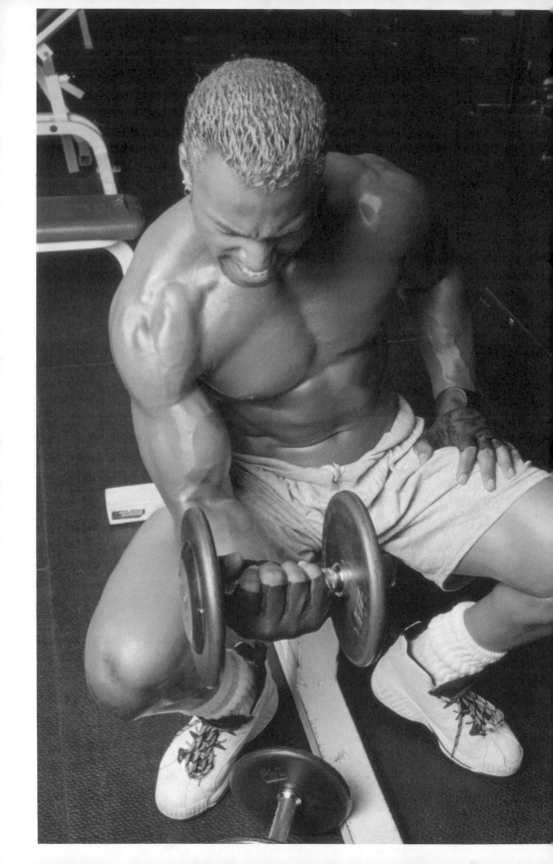

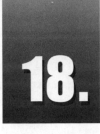

18.

ALTERNATE THE SPEED OF YOUR REPETITIONS

Another way to build mass is to alternate the speed of your repetitions. Super-slow reps increase the demands on the muscle fibers by lengthening the amount of time you spend in the exercise movement. Alternating super-slow reps with the more usual rep speed provides a wider range of stimulation that the muscle must adapt to.

In their quest to build muscle, most athletes focus on the amount of weight they lift and the number of sets and repetitions they do. There is, however, another variable that needs to be taken into consideration: the speed of your repetitions.

Athletes usually perform their repetitions with a relatively explosive movement during the concentric phase of an exercise, which is when the muscle fibers become shorter. They then return to the starting position with a slower motion. This second part of the movement, during which the muscle fibers are lengthening, is called the eccentric phase. This technique can promote significant growth, provided that it is done correctly. The rapid contractions during the concentric phase build power and speed, while the "negatives" done during the eccentric phase place a different type of demand on the muscle as it resists the fall of the weight. However, you can't rely exclusively on this technique if you want to pack on maximum size.

When athletes reduce the speed of their repetitions, they usually increase the amount of time devoted to the eccentric phase. This can cause problems, however, because eccentric movements produce greater delayed muscle soreness than concentric movements. During a negative, fewer fibers are recruited for a particular muscular effort. This increases the tension produced per fiber, resulting in relatively greater microcellular damage to each individual fiber. A marked increase in the levels of certain muscle enzymes has also been noted in the blood after eccentric exercise, confirming that damage to the fibers has taken place. Excessive amounts of eccentric movements can even reduce the level of growth hormone produced. So prolonged negatives are definitely not the way to slow your repetition speed.

A better alternative is to reduce the speed of your concentric movement. Instead of contracting the muscle as quickly as possible, slow the motion down. Start out by taking four seconds to lift the weight, then increase this time over several weeks until you take eight or even ten seconds to fully contract the muscle. This may seem like a minor modification, but try it sometime. Keeping the target muscle under tension for a longer period significantly increases the difficulty of the movement. At a bare minimum, the number of repetitions you do will drop. And if your new rep count is less than six, you will need to temporarily lower the weight you use. But don't despair. In time, your strength will increase enough to allow you to use your old weight again. Eventually, you will be able to add more weight. The slower rep speed also reduces momentum, which allows you to train safely at a very high intensity.

These super-slow reps are a better intensity variation than the old reliance on negatives. Dr. Richard Winett, editor of *Master Trainer,* calls super-slow reps "the most effective intensity builder I have ever tried." You will find that this technique enhances your growth while producing less delayed muscle soreness than traditional negatives. It may seem a bit odd at first to do your repetitions in slow motion, but larger muscle mass will be the welcome result.

KEEP A TRAINING JOURNAL

A training journal gives you a valuable record of each workout. Set aside a space for each bodypart, then write down the number of sets and repetitions you do on each exercise. Also, keep track of the length of your workouts. A journal allows you to appreciate the subtle changes in strength that occur over time. It also increases your motivation as you see these improvements and commit yourself to even-greater intensity in the future.

A training journal can make a major difference in your training progress if you use it correctly. A journal helps you to keep track of your performance on a day-to-day basis and maintains your training on its proper course. When the amount of weight you lift or the number of repetitions goes up, you get instant positive feedback. Without a training record, it is virtually impossible to remember and appreciate all of the subtle changes that occur in your training regimen over time.

Your journal does not have to be a fancy notebook. Any piece of paper will do. There are inexpensive spiral notebooks that can be turned into training journals with the addition of a few lines. (You can even store your pencil in the spiral!) Be sure to write down the length of each workout. As was noted earlier, you can increase the intensity of your training by reducing the rest time between sets. When you record the amount of time between your first and last sets, you give yourself another tool to measure your intensity level.

Set aside a space for each bodypart. Then write down the exercises you do, the order you do them in, the amount of weight you lift and the number of sets and repetitions. You will, of course, be stronger on the first exercise you perform, but you don't have to do exercises in the same order all of the time. Just make sure you increase either the weight or the number of repetitions compared with what you did the last time you performed the exercise in that order. This will ensure progressive resistance on an ongoing basis.

A training journal can help you select the type of exercise program that works best for you. By showing how you respond to a particular program, a training record can establish whether a new program is better for your purposes than the one you were using previously. For example, did adding more sets increase your strength and mass gains, or did it push you into overtraining so the improvements actually slowed down? Without a journal it is very difficult to make an accurate decision, since it's virtually impossible to remember what you lifted on a particular exercise three or four months ago (the minimum amount of time you should take before making a judgement on exercise programs).

A training journal can also be a valuable motivational tool. You can see in black and white all of the progress you have made. This can be important in the long haul, because we never grow as rapidly as we would like. Sometimes, in fact, the progress may seem so slow that you think you're treading water. One look at your training journal may reveal, however, that your strength has increased significantly over the past few months. It just happened so slowly that you weren't aware of it. A training journal can recharge your workouts as you celebrate the gains you have made. The recognition that you have gained strength in the past will inspire you to make additional gains in the future. The past is prologue, as they say. A training journal can help you on your way.

20.

SAFETY FIRST

You can't train while you're injured. Be sure to ask for a spot if there is the slightest doubt in your mind about your ability to do a lift. Don't hold your breath during a repetition, as this raises your blood pressure. Instead, breathe in during the eccentric (negative) movement and force the air out on the concentric movement. Use proper exercise technique all of the time.

Safety doesn't always make it on a list of training principles, but it is fundamental to success. You can't work out when you're injured. A safe-and-sound approach to training will ensure that you continue on an upward path toward the achievement of your goals. In the long run, this is better than impulsively jumping into something before you are ready or trying to lift too much weight to impress someone. Safety comes first, in this and all things.

Athletes tend to be impulsive go-getters. The concepts of patience and safety do not come easily. You need to harness your energy and enthusiasm so it is channeled into constructive ends.

By accepting that muscle growth is a gradual yet long-lasting process, you can fight off the impulses to do more than it is safe to do on a particular day. Of course, you need to push the limits of your abilities. Still, a wise athlete knows the fine line between positive intensity and foolishly going over the edge, and stops just short of that line.

If you have any doubt about your ability to lift a weight, ask a gym-mate for a spot. There is nothing negative about realizing you need assistance and asking for it, especially when it allows you to force out a few more growth-stimulating repetitions. Nearly everyone in a gym will be glad to spot you. They may even ask you to return the favor!

Pay close attention to your breathing. Don't hold your breath while doing an exercise, even involuntarily. Sometimes athletes do this intentionally thinking that it will help their concentration or power, but the opposite is true because the body is deprived of a regular flow of oxygen. The lack of oxygen to the brain, called anoxia, is potentially hazardous. Holding your breath sets off a series of physical changes that results in temporary high blood pressure and forceful heart contractions, especially when heavy weights are used. People have even burst blood vessels in their eyes from the high pressure created. This places needless stress on your heart as well.

Instead of restricting your breathing, use it to your advantage. Think of yourself as a steam engine, and let the forcefulness of your exhaling push your body to new heights of intensity. When you do an eccentric movement, such as going down for a squat or lowering your arms for another biceps curl, breathe in. Then, as you do your concentric movement, such as curling or pushing up from your squat, force the air out while you do your repetition. This will improve your intensity and be a lot safer.

Use proper form on all exercises. Prevent injuries by lifting and lowering the weight without swinging or momentum, and make sure that the weights you lift are within your current capabilities. This will ensure a safe completion of the lift and permit the maximum use of the muscle you are training. It will also produce the greatest growth in the long term.

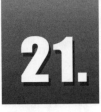

SOCIALIZE BEFORE OR AFTER YOUR WORKOUTS

You're in the gym for one main reason: to build muscle. While socializing is a valuable part of life, there is a time and place for everything. Talk with people before or after your workouts. You could also chat between bodyparts, but don't hold long conversations between sets. Your real friends will understand. Peak concentration and focus will help you achieve your goals as quickly as possible.

Gyms can be great places to meet people. Unlike bars with their smoke and late hours, gyms allow you to connect with healthy men and women who have the same interests you do. Sharing a passion for fitness is an excellent foundation for a relationship, and many people have found that this common bond can lead to long-lasting friendships or even a life partner. Yet, there is a time and place for everything. Socializing at the gym is fine, but don't let it interfere with your workout. The main reason you are at the gym is to grow, so organize your time there in a way that will build as much muscle as possible.

Intensity is a pivotal factor in muscle growth. You need to keep your intensity level high while you do the sets of your bodypart workout. This can be achieved in many ways, including visualization, reducing the time between sets, and the other recommendations in this book. However, you can't achieve peak intensity when you spend five or ten minutes chatting between each set. You could, of course, say a few words during the minute or two while you recuperate between sets, and there is nothing wrong with this as long as you can maintain your mental intensity. Yet, when you lose concentration due to your socializing, you deny yourself an opportunity to grow.

If you want to talk with someone, try to have your conversation before or after your workout. When this isn't possible, at least chat between your bodypart workouts. These recommendations may seem rather restrictive, but you'll find that your real friends will be supportive. They know about your desire to build mass, and they probably share that desire. By channeling your socializing into times that don't interfere with your muscular development, you and your friends can grow together. The extra muscle you gain from your more intense workouts will come in handy when you see someone new at the gym you want to meet!

22.

ACCEPT YOUR GENETICS AND WORK WITH THEM

There are a number of genetic factors that influence muscle growth. Your body type impacts your ability to add size. There also appears to be a genetically set limit in the muscle mass that you can achieve, although many environmental and mental factors influence your success. Accept your genetic profile and tailor your workout to your body's ability to recuperate and grow.

Muscular development is influenced by a number of factors. Many of these are the same for all humans. Others, such as the proportion of fast-twitch and slow-twitch muscle fibers, vary with the individual and are genetically determined. While all humans can improve their muscle growth with weight training, there are certain restraints that genetics places on your size potential.

One of the main genetically determined factors is body structure. There are three main body types: ectomorphs, mesomorphs, and endomorphs. These body types result from the relatively greater growth of particular layers of the embryo before birth.

Ectomorphs are slender in appearance and have difficulty putting on muscle mass. Endomorphs, on the other hand, have thick bones, tend to be heavy and are sometimes fat. They can easily put on body size but find it difficult to lose weight. The mesomorphs are in the middle with moderate bone structures and muscular physiques. Many top bodybuilders are mesomorphs, while basketball players tend to be ectomorphs. Yet, while only three theoretical body structures exist, most athletes are a blend of all three types, with variations in the levels of dominance.

There appears to be a genetically set limit in the muscle mass that an individual can achieve, although it's far greater than what most people imagine. Once the person reaches this point, no amount of training will increase the size of the muscle. This doesn't mean you should stop working out, however. Continued training is necessary to maintain this peak muscle mass. Exercise also provides many other psychological and health benefits, all of which are independent of body size. Training (especially aerobic training) helps reduce body fat as well, so the muscles are more visible.

A person's maximum growth potential is determined by their genetics to a significant degree. This is a fact of life. Our muscle-fiber compositions vary, as do our cardiovascular capabilities, natural hormone levels and points of muscle insertion. Our abilities to recuperate also vary. These factors can limit your ability to respond to exercise. Some people's muscles seem to grow from just a few months of training, while others train for a year or more to get similar results.

At the same time, there are many environmental and mental factors that influence muscular development. These include the determination to keep to a training schedule, the ability to react positively to the physical and psychological pressures of competition, and the capacity to push through the pain barrier during training. Your diet and the amount of sleep you get are under your control, too. All of these factors will impact your success.

Your age also influences your ability to grow, although scientists have found that age is a much less important factor than originally thought. What was once considered an inevitable decline in muscle size now turns out to be dependent on environmental and lifestyle factors such as diet and exercise. Athletes can build muscle in their eighties if the desire is there. While they might not out-perform a teenager, they will nonetheless enhance their quality of life and feel the exercise "high" from all those wonderful endorphins rushing through their systems.

There is no question that genetics plays a major role in muscular development. Some athletes simply have the ability to achieve greater muscle mass than others. But don't give up and become a couch potato. Accept your genetics and work with them. Tailor your workout program to your body's ability to recuperate and grow. Don't train yourself into the ground just because you see other people doing it. Follow your own path. Respect the signals that your body gives you and it will respond with the greatest muscle growth your genetics allow. Regardless of your ultimate mass potential, sports activity will improve the quality of your life. The satisfaction you get along the way will be its own reward.

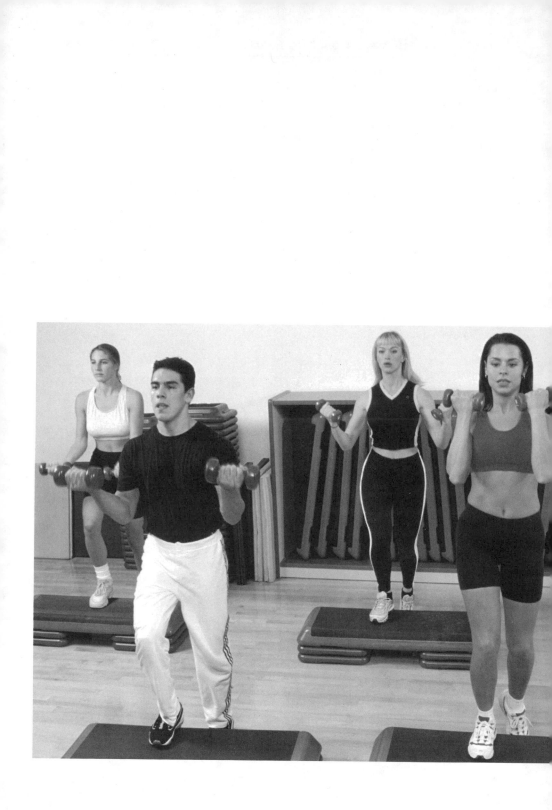

23.

LIMIT THE AMOUNT OF AEROBICS YOU DO

Aerobic exercise is essential for cardiovascular fitness, but you can overdo a good thing. Studies have shown that too much aerobic activity can reduce your gains in strength and muscle size compared with weight training alone. Restrict your aerobic activities to 1 to $1\frac{1}{2}$ hours per week and vary the type of aerobics you do. Keep your food intake under control, too. You'll have bigger muscles and a more defined physique.

Aerobic exercise is a necessary part of a balanced training program. Aerobic conditioning strengthens the cardiovascular system by forcing the heart to work at elevated rates for a longer period of time than occurs with most weight-training routines. Aerobics helps burn the free fatty acids in the body as well, resulting in a more defined, muscular physique. Moderate amounts of aerobic activity can also stimulate the conversion of lactic acid back into pyruvic acid and glucose, which gives your muscles more fuel for additional contractions.

You can have too much of a good thing, however. A study by

Dr. Kraemer and colleagues at the Center for Sports Medicine at Pennsylvania State University found that strength and power increases declined when an endurance-training program was added to a weight-training regimen. The men who only trained with weights had a 30 percent improvement in their leg-press performance over twelve weeks. Yet, when a four-day-a-week aerobics program was added, a matched group had a performance increase of only 19.5 percent. The researchers also found that endurance training reduced the size of the muscle fibers created by weight training while increasing production of the catabolic hormone, cortisol. "Resistance training increases protein synthesis and the amount of contractile protein in the muscle fiber," notes Dr. Kraemer. "On the other hand, the stress from endurance training causes the muscle to respond in an opposite direction by degrading the contractile proteins to optimize oxygen uptake. The end result was a reduction in the athletes' strength and muscle gains."

Therefore, you need to control the amount of aerobics you do. One to one-and-a-half hours per week is all you really need to keep your cardiovascular system in good working order. This aerobic conditioning should consist of two or three thirty- to forty-five-minute sessions. Be sure to do at least a half-hour of aerobics at any one time because it takes a while for your body to switch into the aerobic (fat-burning) energy system. Too short of an exercise session will therefore not provide you with all of the desired benefits. Remember to include a five-minute warm-up and a five-minute cool-down with your aerobics as well as a bit of stretching. Don't count this time as part of your minimum half-hour, however.

Pace yourself so that your aerobics is as beneficial as possible. Try to do your aerobic activity at an intensity level that is from 60 to 80 percent of your maximum heart rate. Much more than 80 percent will increase the involvement of the body's other energy systems, and anything less than 60 percent will be so low that you'll need to spend a lot more time exercising to burn the fat you want to get rid of. It's also less exercise for your heart. To determine your maximum heart rate per minute, subtract your age from 220. (Your maximum rate declines with age.) Then multiply that rate by 60 and 80 percent to determine your desired range of heartbeats. You can measure your heart rate by taking your pulse manually or with one of the machines now on the market.

Also, make it a point to vary the aerobic activities you do. The body is a very efficient mechanism, and it responds to changes in its environment by adapting to the demands placed on it. Simply put, if all you do for aerobics is jog, your body will get very efficient at that activity. This is a great way to conserve energy, but nowadays most people are more concerned with limiting their body-fat levels. Stationary or outdoor bicycling, rowing machine, skiing machine, in-line skating, stair climbing, and powerwalking are all excellent ways to work your heart. These variations will also make your aerobic training a lot more interesting.

If you find that your legs get sore from aerobics and remain sore until you plan to weight train your legs, cut back on the volume of aerobics or weight training or both. Your legs can't grow if they are constantly sustaining microcellular damage. They need an opportunity to recuperate and establish a foundation for future growth. You could also change the type of aerobics you do. Rowing machines and swimming utilize the upper body as well as the legs, reducing the relative energy requirement for the legs. If you place too many demands on your legs, their growth will slow down or stop altogether.

You can also get cardiovascular benefits from your weight training when you rest a short time between sets. A six-week study by Petersen at the University of Alberta measured the maximum volume of oxygen that weight-training football players and rowers could utilize at their peak capacity (VO_2 max). The researchers noted a 8 percent increase in VO_2 max when the athletes maintained a work-to-rest ratio of 1:2, along with an equivalent gain in maximal stroke volume (the greatest amount of blood that the heart can pump in a single beat). A similar study by Gettman found a 8 percent increase in VO_2 max when the time between sets was 30 seconds and a 12 percent improvement with a 15-second break between sets.

While this is less rest than most athletes are used to, it appears to be necessary to improve cardiovascular fitness because the heart rate remains elevated throughout the entire workout. On the bright side, this can reduce the amount of traditional aerobic activity that you need to do each week. You may find, however, that you aren't able to fully recover from your previous set with such short breaks, so the muscle's strength level may suffer.

Experiment to see which work-to-rest ratio is best for you. As was noted in Chapter 8, there are numerous benefits when you reduce the time between sets. And if you can get a cardiovascular benefit as well, all the better. Just don't let it negatively impact your long-term strength levels. They are essential to packing on more muscle mass.

Body fat is nothing more than energy that has been consumed but not utilized by the body. You should regulate your food intake so that it approximates your energy expenditure. This is the most efficient method for the body, and it also minimizes the amount of time required for your aerobic training program. It is pointless to overeat and then spend hours on the treadmill or stationary bike to burn off the excess. Try to maintain a diet that provides enough nutrients for muscle growth but not much more. This way you'll have a healthier heart and look great year round!

Part Two

DIET AND SUPPLEMENTATION

INTRODUCTION

The adage that you are what you eat is particularly true for athletes. You push your body to the limit in order to build muscle mass and excel in your chosen sport. This intense activity puts significant demands on the body. Not only must you consume enough food to provide the energy needed for your active lifestyle, but you have to give your body the nutrients required to recuperate from the stresses of training. When you give your body what it needs and wants, it responds by letting your muscles grow bigger and stronger.

On the other hand, without the proper balance and quantities of nutrients, you could train until the cows come home and not see favorable results from your workouts. Progressive resistance training is an essential element in your program for achieving muscle growth, but it is only part of the equation. To build your ideal physique as quickly as possible, you need to take the time to buy and consume the right types of foods and supplements. If you devote part of your daily energy to this important task, you will find that your body returns the favor by giving you a new spurt of muscle growth.

Part Two focuses on thirteen different aspects of sports nutrition. The three macronutrients (protein, carbohydrates, and fats) are first discussed so you can understand their individual roles and see how they interact within the body's metabolic pathways. A variety of dietary tips are then offered ranging from meal frequency and water consumption to the role of splurges. The need for supplementation is also explored, and a number of recommendations are made for vitamins, minerals, and several sports nutrients. Part Two concludes with a discussion of how you can tailor your supplement program to your particular needs and budget. Let's see how you can get the most benefit from the foods and nutrients you eat.

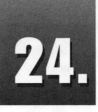

EAT PLENTY
OF PROTEIN

Protein is vitally important for muscle growth. There are thousands of different proteins in the body, and all are made directly or indirectly from the amino acids in the foods and supplements we eat. Athletes need much more than the Recommended Dietary Allowance (RDA) of protein. Most strength athletes should eat 0.8 grams of protein per pound of bodyweight each day. Endurance athletes need 0.6 grams per pound of bodyweight daily. Divide this protein requirement into four to five equal portions.

Protein is an essential nutrient for athletes. There is some protein in every single cell of the human body. Brain cells, for example, are 10 percent protein while red blood cells and muscle cells contain as much as 20 percent protein. All in all, protein makes up nearly 15 percent of a person's bodyweight, more than any other substance except water. These proteins have a wide range of functions, including tissue growth and development. Two protein-based myofilaments inside the muscle fiber, known as actin and myosin, are responsible for all muscle contraction. The tendons, ligaments, hair, skin, and nails are specialized kinds of structural proteins. Proteins are also used to form some two thousand different enzymes, which speed up chemical reactions throughout the body. Proteins are even needed to form most hormones, including insulin and growth hormone.

The body manufactures all of these different proteins directly or indirectly from the raw materials in the proteins you eat. These building blocks are called amino acids. There are twenty amino acids in foods: alanine, arginine, asparagine, aspartic acid, cysteine, glutamine, glutamic acid, glycine, histidine, isoleucine, leucine, lysine, methionine, phenylalanine, proline, serine, threonine, tryptophan, tyrosine, and valine. All of these amino acids contain nitrogen and other components. When the body has enough of them, it is said to have a positive nitrogen balance. Inadequate protein consumption relative to your needs results in a negative nitrogen balance.

The adult body can manufacture twelve of these amino acids whenever they are needed. They are called nonessential amino acids. This does not mean they are unimportant, however. The term nonessential signifies that the body can synthesize them from compounds normally present in the body at a rate equal to the body's need for them. The other eight amino acids are called essential because they must be supplied by the diet. These essential amino acids are isoleucine, leucine, lysine, methionine, phenylalanine, threonine, tryptophan, and valine.

Foods are classified by the quality of the amino acids in them. Complete proteins are foods that contain amino acids in the correct quantities and ratios to support tissue growth and repair. Eating the right amount of these foods assures you an adequate supply of all of the essential amino acids. Incomplete proteins, on the other hand, are those foods that lack enough of one or more of the essential amino acids. When incomplete proteins are eaten as the protein source, it is possible to have a protein deficiency even if the total quantity of protein eaten is sufficient for your needs. This is because the deficient amino acid becomes a limiting factor for the protein production process, effectively stopping protein synthesis even though all of the other amino acids are available in adequate quantities.

As a result, athletes must consume complete proteins. You can do this by eating proteins that are complete by themselves or by eating two protein sources that together contain all of the essential amino acids. Foods that are individually complete include eggs, milk, meat, fish, and poultry. Whole eggs have the best combination of essential amino acids among unprocessed foods. They have therefore been used as the foundation for a protein measurement system called Biologic Value. As can be seen in Table 24.1, whole eggs have a Biologic Value of 100. Milk is ranked at 91, while whey protein tops the chart at 104. Most meats are around 80. Vegetable sources of protein rank even lower because they lack certain essential amino acids.

It is also possible to get adequate protein from vegetable products if the foods are eaten in the right combinations. Basically, beans or nuts should be eaten with grains like corn, wheat, or rice. Tofu, which is made from soybeans, should also be eaten with grains. These combinations create complete protein foods by combining one food that is deficient in a particular amino acid with another food that contains it. Complementary foods should be eaten within a few hours of each other.

One of the main questions that athletes ask is how much protein they should consume. The U.S. Government has established a Recommended Dietary Allowance (RDA) of 0.8 grams per kilogram (g/kg) of bodyweight per day. That's equal to 0.36 grams per

Table 24.1. Biologic Values

Protein Source	Biologic Value	Protein Source	Biologic Value
Whey	104	Soy	74
Egg, whole	100	Rice	59
Milk	91	Wheat	54
Egg white	88	Peanuts	43
Beef	80	Dry Beans	34
Fish	78	Potato	34
Casein	77		

pound (g/lb). While some nutritionists maintain that this is a liberal allowance that provides enough protein for active individuals, most athletes feel that the body's demand for protein increases significantly due to training. Recent research has backed them up.

"Athletes break down their muscle tissue during training, so they need more protein than sedentary individuals to rebuild it and get a growth response," notes Dr. Mauro Di Pasquale of the University of Toronto. "Protein can also be used for energy, particularly during endurance activities and weight-loss programs." "Synthesizing new muscle tissue requires the building blocks of amino acids and sufficient energy (calorie) intake," adds Dr. Pete Lemon of the University of Western Ontario. "New research has confirmed what athletes have said for 100 years: consuming only the RDA of protein can actually hold back your progress."

Using nitrogen balance analysis and advanced metabolic tracers, scientists have determined that athletes with vigorous training schedules can require at least double the RDA to maintain a positive nitrogen balance. Pete Lemon and associates found that strength athletes need 1.7 to 1.8 g/kg (about 0.8 g/lb). Endurance athletes need a bit less: 1.2 to 1.4 g/kg (about 0.6 g/lb). These figures are based on total bodyweight. Although body fat does not require protein, this makes it easier for athletes to compute their protein requirements. Using these guidelines, a 200-pound strength athlete would need around 160 grams of protein daily. A 200-pound endurance athlete would require about 120 grams of high quality protein per day.

A study by Fern suggests that there is an upper limit to the amount of protein you can use. This experiment compared a group of men who consumed 1.3 g/kg/day of protein with a group that ate 3.3 g/kg/day for five weeks. During four of these weeks, the study participants performed strength-training exercises. The group that ate more protein had greater nitrogen retention and larger increases in muscle size. The 3.3 g/kg group gained an average of 6 pounds of lean body mass, while the athletes consuming 1.3 g/kg gained only half as much muscle during the month. However, Fern also discovered that the 3.3 g/kg group had 2.5 times more urinary nitrogen excretion and a 159-percent increase in protein oxidation. Basically, a significant amount of the additional protein either wound up in these athletes' urine or was broken down into carbohydrate or fat and not used to directly build muscle. "There is a ceiling effect on protein consumption," notes Dr. Lemon. "If you eat more than you need, the excess will just be wasted." You can have too much of a good thing!

Bodybuilders and other strength athletes who train at very high weight loads, volumes, and exercise intensities may need more protein than other athletes. "As you increase the demands on your body, your protein requirements increase proportionally," says Dr. Di Pasquale, who is author of the excellent reference book *Amino Acids and Proteins for the Athlete: The Anabolic Edge*. "It has been my experience that some athletes need as much as 1.1 g/lb (2.5 g/kg) to achieve the greatest muscle growth." Unfortunately, the study that would definitively prove this is still in the proposal stage. If you are an athlete who trains with very high weights, volumes, or intensities, you may wish to experiment with this higher protein intake to see whether you experience an incremental boost in strength or mass. However, for the vast majority of male and female athletes, the basic protein dosages recommended in this book will provide sufficient protein for your muscle development.

You need to eat an adequate amount of complete protein every day, even on the days you don't exercise. The body uses protein continuously to provide the raw materials for muscle growth, repair and maintenance. Only so much protein can be stored inside the cells and in the blood's free amino acid pool. When you consume too much at once, the body eventually converts the excess into carbohydrate or fat through a complex process. Your muscles need a continuous supply of amino acids to achieve their optimal growth, so you should give them what they want when they want it. At the same time, there is no scientific evidence to support the frequently heard idea that the body can only assimilate 35 grams of protein at once. Eat more than this amount per meal if you like, but don't try to consume all of your protein at two or three meals if at all possible.

You can wind up with a negative nitrogen balance even at the recommended protein levels if you do not consume enough carbohydrates as well. This can occur during the carbohydrate-depletion diets that are sometimes used prior to competitions with weight classes. It often occurs during long-distance marathon racing, too. When your body needs energy and does not have sufficient carbohydrates to meet its needs, it uses up all of the glycogen (stored glucose) it has available and then converts the protein in its liver and muscle stores into energy. This can result in a loss in muscle mass, as the body literally eats away at itself to provide the nutrients it needs. Hardly what an athlete wants!

You may have heard that excessive protein consumption stresses the kidneys. However, there is no published evidence that the high protein intakes consumed by many athletes leads to kidney disease. In fact, a study by Zaragoza observed only minimal alterations to kidney function when he gave rodents a diet that was 80 percent protein for more than half their life spans. Still, protein foods are much more expensive than carbohydrates and fats, so it is pointless to eat more than you have to. Also, a 1997 study by Volek found that high protein consumption reduces testosterone levels at rest compared with a diet with less protein and relatively more carbohydrates. So not only do you waste money by eating too much protein, you can actually lower the supply of one of your main anabolic hormones.

In the last decade, a wide variety of protein supplements have become available. These soy, milk and egg, and whey powders have their own unique advantages and disadvantages. You need to be a smart shopper to select the supplement with the best cost/benefit ratio for you.

Soy powders were the first protein powders on the market. Initially they had a chalky taste and were not well refined. Newer soy blends are of much better taste and quality and can be as high as 99-percent protein. They also come in a variety of flavors and have the advantage of being the least expensive powders. However, because it is a vegetable protein, soy has a number of special characteristics. "Soy powders are low in methionine," notes Dr. Di Pasquale, "although soy has a higher glutamine content than whey. It is also high in branched-chain amino acids and arginine, both of which are important for muscle growth. Yet, some of the isoflavonoids in soy exert an estrogenic effect, which can be counterproductive for male athletes." Many soy products require a blender too, although the newer, top-of-the-line products are easier to mix.

Milk and egg powders contain casein, whey, and egg whites in varying proportions. As cheese is produced, the milk divides into two main products: a solid portion called casein and a liquid known as whey. Since whey was considered a waste product until recently, most of the milk and egg powders are predominantly casein with smaller amounts of egg white and whey. "Casein slows down the transport of amino acids in the gut, which increases their absorption," says Di Pasquale. "It also has greater amounts of the amino acids that can be used for energy during exercise." However, milk and egg powders are hard to dissolve, so you need to use a blender. They cost more than soy products, but are less expensive than whey. Because casein contains lactose, it can cause gastrointestinal disturbances in some individuals.

Whey powders have been all the rage during the last few years. In the early part of this decade, scientists developed a number of systems to distill the whey into a high-quality powder that is also fat- and lactose-free. These ion-exchange and microfiltration systems use cool temperatures that preserve the taste and natural configurations of the amino acids. Whey has the highest Biologic Value of any protein. It dissolves easily in water, allowing the athlete to mix a protein drink on the run. However, whey has less glutamine, arginine, and phenylalanine than either casein or soy. It can also cost significantly more than these other proteins. While whey products that use the old high-temperature process cost less, they are not as effective because the proteins are denatured and less biologically active.

Every type of protein powder has its own unique characteristics. By combining the different powders together, you could get a broad-based spectrum of amino acids that eliminates the comparative disadvantages of each. Remember, however, that these supplements are not intended to replace the protein in your regular meals. Their value lies in giving you an easy way to get additional protein when your meals do not provide enough to meet your daily requirement. Supplementation can therefore ensure that you get all of the amino acids you need for your exercise program, helping you to achieve the goals you have set for your sport.

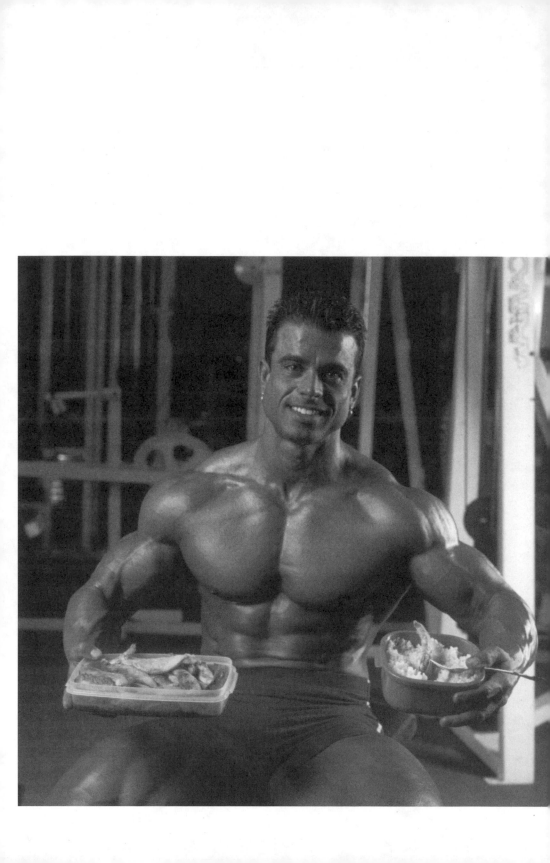

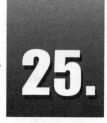

25.

CONSUME CARBOHYDRATES WITH A LOW GLYCEMIC INDEX

Adequate carbohydrate intake is essential. Carbs are converted to glucose, which is the body's preferred source of fuel. Some carbohydrates are assimilated more quickly than others. You should mainly eat carbs with a low glycemic index, such as pasta, beans, vegetables and fruits. An intake of 2 to 3 grams per pound of bodyweight is sufficient for most athletes. If you are restricting your carb intake to "make weight" for a competition, add psyllium to your diet.

Carbohydrates are the best source of energy fuel for the body. Although proteins can be converted into energy, the calories in carbohydrate foods offer the most efficient and least taxing way for the body to get the energy it needs. The brain and central nervous system rely on the carbohydrate glucose to function normally. Carbohydrates also provide part of the energy for muscular contraction, particularly during weightlifting and other high-intensity activities. An adequate level of carbohydrates in the diet allows all of the dietary protein you consume to be used for its primary purpose of tissue growth and development. For this reason, carbohydrates are said to have a protein-sparing effect. A diet that is high in carbohydrates will also be relatively low in fats, which helps to prevent heart disease and other health problems.

Even though the muscles and liver can store about half a pound (400 to 500 g) of glucose as glycogen, this limited capacity can be depleted by only a few hours of training, depending on your sport and intensity level. When glycogen stores are used up, fatigue sets in and exercise must stop. Marathon runners call this "hitting the wall." It is therefore essential that an adequate supply of carbohydrates be available at all times for maximum performance.

Carbohydrates are needed to fully process dietary fats for energy. The body only partially metabolizes fats if insufficient carbohydrates are available, which results in an acidic condition known as ketosis. The body can literally run out of fuel even if fat calories are theoretically available. This explains how "zero-carb" diets (when only fats and proteins are consumed) can cause athletes to run out of energy and feel "brain-dead" even when eating a moderate level of non-carbohydrate calories. If you have ever considered doing a zero-carb diet to make weight for a competition, forget it. This diet can actually lead to fat retention as the body's protective mechanisms respond to what they perceive as starvation. Hypoglycemia and its accompanying dizziness, hunger, and weakness can also occur. The best way to lose fat is to continue eating some carbohydrates and slowly reduce your total caloric intake while continuing your exercise program.

It was once felt that all simple sugars were digested and assimilated rapidly by the body, producing a large increase in blood-sugar levels and soon afterward a rise in insulin secretion. Complex carbohydrates, on the other hand, were thought to assimilate more slowly, resulting in less rapid changes in blood-sugar and insulin levels. Research has shown that this view of digestion and assimilation is too simplistic.

While there is a great deal of variation in the time it takes for particular foods to be absorbed into the bloodstream, factors other than the structure of the sugar are often involved. Table 25.1 lists the glycemic index for many common foods. As you can see, some sugary products, like a candy bar, are actually converted into blood glucose at a rate slower than potatoes. Rice can cause a greater rise in blood sugar than fruits such as apples and oranges, while pure fructose will stimulate less insulin production than spaghetti. Foods that contain fat are assimilated more slowly than pure carbohydrate foods.

Table 25.1. Glycemic Index for Selected Foods

Food	Glycemic Index	Food	Glycemic Index
BREAKFAST CEREALS		**LEGUMES**	
All-bran	51	Beans, baked	40
Cornflakes	80	Beans, butter	36
Oatmeal	54	Beans, kidney	29
Shredded Wheat	67	Chick-peas	36
		Green peas	51
DAIRY PRODUCTS		Lentils	29
Ice cream	36	Soybeans	15
Milk, skim	32		
Milk, whole	34	**MISCELLANEOUS**	
Yogurt	36	Candy bar	68
		Honey	87
FRUITS		Peanuts	13
Apples	39	Potato chips	51
Bananas	62		
Oranges	40	**SUGARS**	
Orange juice	46	Fructose	20
Raisins	64	Glucose	100
		Maltose	105
GRAINS		Sucrose	59
Bread, wheat	72		
Bread, white	69	**VEGETABLES**	
Rice, brown	66	Beets	64
Rice, white	72	Carrots	92
Spaghetti, wheat	42	Corn on cob	59
Spaghetti, white	50	Potato	70
		Yam	51

The glycemic index can be of great value to athletes who are loading up on carbohydrates for a competition. Since foods with a lower glycemic index are assimilated at a slower rate, they can provide a more steady supply of energy than the higher glycemic index foods, which are more likely to provide the "sugar rush" and "sugar down" associated with sweets. Lower-index foods will also result in higher muscle-glycogen levels and less storage of the glucose as fat. While the glycemic index of each food changes when they are mixed together in a meal, it is always a good idea to get the bulk of your calories from grains, beans, vegetables, and fruits due to their greater nutritional and fiber content. Of course, everyone has cravings for sweets once in a while. Just try to make these splurges the exception and not the rule.

Sometimes athletes go without fruit for extended periods before a competition, thinking that it is a simple sugar. Yet, they may eat so much steamed rice and plain baked potato that they feel it may start coming out of their ears. One look at the glycemic index shows that there is no point to this dietary hardship. Fruits are actually assimilated more slowly than rice and potatoes due to their greater fiber content. A piece of fruit will not hold back your sports progress, and it will make your diet easier to tolerate.

You should eat a relatively constant supply of carbohydrates each day. Depending on your exercise intensity and the speed of your metabolism, 2 to 3 g of carbs per pound of bodyweight (4.5 to 6.5 g/kg) should permit full restoration of your glycogen stores without an accumulation of bodyfat. Endurance athletes and strength athletes on high-volume training regimens may need more than this amount. Also, be sure to spread out your carbohydrate consumption. The best way to maintain a relatively constant blood-glucose level is to eat carbs throughout the day. Because the body has a significant storage capacity for glucose in its glycogen stores, this is not as important as the regular consumption of protein. Still, you should never avoid carbs during the day and then stuff yourself at dinner.

Many carbohydrates have fiber, which is a component of plant foods that cannot be assimilated by the human digestive system. There are actually two types of fiber: soluble and insoluble. Soluble fiber is capable of absorbing many times its weight in water in the stomach and intestines. It also binds with the cholesterol-based bile acids that are secreted by the liver, resulting in a lower level of cholesterol in the blood. Insoluble fiber, on the other hand, doesn't absorb much of anything. It does, however, add bulk to the stool, which has a gentle, scrubbing action that helps cleanse the walls of the bowel.

People that eat large amounts of vegetables, fruits, and whole-grain products usually get enough fiber in their diets. However, athletes who are competing in an event with weight classes sometimes cut back on their consumption of carbohydrates even though they continue to eat large amounts of protein. While this reduces their caloric intake, it also lowers their fiber consumption and may negatively affect their cholesterol count, although many factors can influence your cholesterol level.

One way to keep your fiber intake up is to add a tablespoon of psyllium to your cereal and to protein shakes. Unflavored psyllium is sold at many health food and drug stores. It has no digestible calories and 7 g of fiber per tablespoon. Psyllium won't directly improve muscle growth, but it will help keep your cardiovascular system in good working order. And your heart is the most important muscle of all.

Athletes sometimes feel guilty about eating carbs. Their desire to have a lean, muscular physique can lead them to avoid carbohydrates and then consume vast quantities of protein. This places pointless stress on the body. Remember that your muscles can't be "pumped to the max" unless your glycogen stores are filled to the brim. It's all a matter of degree. Too many carbs, of course, will result in stored body fat, but too few carbs will hold back your progress. So give your muscles their preferred source of fuel in just the right amounts for growth. You could be pleasantly surprised with the results.

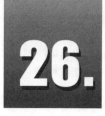

26.

KEEP YOUR FAT INTAKE LOW

Your body needs a small amount of two essential fatty acids each day: linoleic and linolenic acids. Flaxseed oil is an excellent source of these acids, although they are found in smaller amounts in fish and other fatty foods. A diet that is 10- to 15-percent fat usually provides enough of these nutrients. Depending on your workout program and metabolism, greater fat intake may result in bodyfat accumulation without any corresponding sports benefit.

Dietary fat is one of the most misunderstood aspects of sports nutrition. The traditional American diet contains very high levels of fat, far more than can be justified from a health perspective. Even today, the average American consumes over 40 percent of his or her total calories in the form of fat. On the other hand, some athletes have concluded that all fats are bad, leading to diets that eliminate virtually all sources of this nutrient. The truth lies in between.

Fat actually has a number of vital functions in the body. It is needed to absorb vitamins A, D, E, and K. Fat also contains linoleic and linolenic acids, two essential fatty acids that are every bit as important for good nutrition as the essential amino acids. Linoleic and linolenic acid must be supplied by the diet, yet not all fatty foods contain them in large amounts. In addition to supplying the body with energy, these fatty acids are components of our cellular membranes and nerve cells. They also assist in the growth process and are part of hormone-like substances known as prostaglandins.

Fat also serves as the body's long-term energy source, providing energy for all tissues of the body except the brain, nerves, and lungs. Since the body has only a limited capacity to store carbohydrates and proteins, all nutrients that are not immediately needed for energy or anabolic activities are converted to fat and stored in the adipose tissues for later use. This allows the body to maintain its normal functioning between meals.

The fat stores are an important energy source during light and moderate exercise. During long periods of jogging, up to 80 percent of the energy produced comes from the fat stores. That is why it is so important to include aerobic activities in a program of weight reduction. At the same time, anaerobic sports such as weightlifting and sprinting do not use fats for energy because these activities are so intense and short-term that the body's aerobic energy system cannot be geared up for action quickly enough to be of assistance. Glycogen, glucose, and a compound called ATP (adenosine triphosphate) provide the fuel for these anaerobic activities.

There are three types of fat: saturated, monounsaturated, and polyunsaturated. Mainly saturated fats, such as butter and lard, are solid at room temperature. Meats and cheeses also contain high levels of saturated fat, which raises the amount of cholesterol in the blood and increases the risk of atherosclerosis (hardening of the arteries). Monounsaturated fats, including avocado, olive, canola and peanut oils, are much healthier. They have even been shown to inhibit bodyfat gains in mice compared with mice given an equivalent amount of saturated fat. Polyunsaturated fats are more unsaturated than the monounsaturated fats. Examples of these fats are corn, soybean, and safflower oils.

All sources of fat have a mixture of both saturated and unsaturated fats in them. As a general rule, animal fats are predominately saturated while vegetable oils are mostly unsaturated. There are exceptions, however. Palm kernel and coconut oils are made up of mostly saturated fatty acids, while chicken fat has a great deal of unsaturated fat. Fish oils are also high in polyunsaturated fatty acids. Hydrogenated or partially hydrogenated vegetable oil is actually unsaturated vegetable oil that has been chemically processed to make it more saturated. Products with these modified oils should be avoided for the same reasons you steer away from saturated fats.

High levels of fat consumption have been linked to diabetes, obesity, hypertension and even cancer. They can adversely affect the transport of glucose into skeletal muscle, restricting the formation of the glycogen stores. They can even reduce the effectiveness of insulin and the oxygen-carrying capacity of the blood. For these reasons, it is wise for athletes to restrict the total amount of fat in their diets.

Athletes who are interested in health and maximum strength gains should consume a diet that is 10- to 15-percent fat. This will provide enough of the two essential fatty acids while keeping the impact on your total caloric intake to a minimum. (Fats have nine calories per gram versus four calories for proteins and carbohydrates). Depending on your workout program and metabolism, greater fat intake may result in bodyfat accumulation without any corresponding sports benefit. You could also eat a relatively fat-free diet and consume a tablespoon or two of flaxseed (linseed) oil each day. This oil is an excellent source of linoleic and linolenic acids, which are known as omega-3 and omega-6 fatty acids, respectively. Evening primrose oil and borage oil are also good sources of these fats, but they are much more expensive. Flaxseed oil has relatively more omega-3 acids, while primrose oil and borage oil have higher amounts of omega-6 acids. Cold water fish, such as tuna, and fish-oil supplements also have high amounts of omega-3s.

You can minimize your exposure to saturated fat by eating mostly fish, chicken, turkey, and egg whites for your protein sources. This will keep your total fat intake down as well. Reduce your beef, pork, and egg-yolk consumption to a minimum, and when you eat meat buy a very lean cut and trim away all of the visible fat. Throw out your butter dish and keep on driving past those fast-food restaurants. Over time, these dietary changes will give you a trimmer, more defined physique that will show off the results of your hard work at the gym.

27.

DIVIDE YOUR FOOD INTAKE INTO FOUR OR FIVE MEALS

Muscles require nutrients on a regular basis. In order to pack on mass, you have to give your muscles the proteins, carbohydrates, fats and micronutrients they need to support the growth process throughout the day. Never skip breakfast, and make sure you eat immediately after your workout and again two hours later. Increasing the number of meals from the traditional three to four or five also increases your metabolic rate slightly, which helps to keep your bodyfat level under control.

While the total daily intake of nutrients is an important consideration for muscle growth, the timing of your meals also impacts your gains. In order to achieve the greatest increase in mass, you need to give your body the nutrients it requires when they are most needed. It's not enough to eat a couple of big meals whenever they happen to fit into your schedule. Although two meals a day will permit some improvements, you need to make more of a commitment to your diet if you want to excel at your sport. You have to make the time in your busy day to eat four or five relatively smaller meals. This should include the traditional "three squares" a day plus one or two nutritious snacks. It may take a bit of adjustment at first, but the results are worth the effort.

One reason to divide your food intake into four or five meals is that it moderately increases your basal metabolic rate (BMR) for a while. Your BMR is the number of calories it takes to maintain all of your biological functions without any physical movement on your part. The BMR declines about 30 percent during sleep. When you eat a meal, there is a temporary rise in your BMR. This is called the thermic effect of food. Basically, your body speeds up 5 to 10 percent for an hour or two to process the food ingested. Of course, this thermic effect is not sufficient to burn all of the extra calories in the meal, for if it did no one would be overweight. Yet, when you divide a given number of calories per day into four or five meals, you wind up with less bodyfat than if you had eaten the same amount of food in three meals.

Another way to maximize muscle growth is by creating the ideal hormonal environment. This is achieved by manipulating your meal timing so that the largest amount of insulin, growth hormone and testosterone is secreted during and after your workout. The higher levels of these anabolic hormones will promote more protein synthesis in the muscle fibers and minimize the impact of other catabolic hormones such as cortisol. Insulin enhances growth in part by stimulating amino acid uptake into the muscle cells. As it moves these amino acids and glucose out of the bloodstream, it also creates an environment that results in greater growth hormone secretion later in the day. The uptake of testosterone into the muscle cells also appears to increase. You can maximize these benefits by avoiding food before your workout and by eating two meals after your workout, one immediately after your exercise session and another two hours later. Your other three meals should be eaten at three- to four-hour intervals whenever they are most convenient.

Sometimes athletes feel that they need to eat before a workout in order to have enough energy to perform at their best. However, the predominant energy source for weightlifting is stored glycogen. (A compound called ATP supplies most of your remaining energy needs during muscle contraction.) If you have eaten correctly the day before, you will have enough glycogen in your muscles and liver to give it your all at the gym. In fact, pre-exercise meals can actually hinder your progress. A study by Cappon at Harbor-UCLA Medical Center found that eating a meal with high levels of carbohydrate or fat before a workout substantially reduced post-exercise growth hormone (hGH) secretion. Following an overnight fast, eleven young adults performed high-intensity exercise on a bicycle ergometer after drinking a liquid meal or a placebo. The researchers discovered that the carbohydrate drink reduced hGH levels by 24 percent, while the fat meal caused a 54-percent drop.

Although a pre-workout meal will cause a temporary rise in your insulin levels, so much insulin is secreted that the level of blood-sugar ends up being too low, requiring the release of glucagon to raise the level back to where it should be. During this period of overreaction, your energy level will be lower than normal, not higher. It is better to train on an empty stomach so that your insulin and blood-sugar fluctuations are minimized. This will also allow relatively more free fatty acids to be "burned" for fuel between your sets. This fatty-acid oxidation occurs to the greatest extent during morning workouts.

A number of positive hormonal changes usually occur during a training session. Exercise causes a boost in growth hormone secretion, which not only increases the use of fatty acids for energy but stimulates nitrogen retention and the production of various growth factors as well. Testosterone concentrations also increase in response to exercise. Yet, they too have been shown to decrease when insulin levels are high. It makes no sense to reduce your supply of growth hormone and testosterone while you train by eating before you get to the gym.

A far better option is to eat right after your workout and again two hours later. Two studies have shown that this technique produces the fastest rate of glycogen storage along with beneficial increases in insulin and growth hormone when you need them most. Chandler and associates at the University of Texas at Austin measured the hormonal responses of nine male weightlifters to four different post-workout meals: a carbohydrate meal, a protein meal, a carbohydrate and protein meal, and a placebo (water). The meals were given immediately after their workouts and again in two hours. Chandler found that while the carb meal and protein meal each stimulated a rise in insulin levels, the greatest increase occurred when both carbs and protein were eaten. (Total food intake was kept constant.) This mixed meal also produced the greatest growth hormone levels five to six hours after exercise. Although the blood level of testosterone dropped during this period, the researchers speculated that this was due to an increased uptake of testosterone into the muscles. This would have an anabolic effect by stimulating protein synthesis. A similar experiment by Zawadzki with male cyclists found that the carb/protein meal restored muscle glycogen levels 38-percent faster than the carbohydrate meal alone.

In order to stimulate the greatest hormone responses to exercise, eat 0.5 grams of carbohydrates and 0.25 grams of protein per pound of bodyweight after your workout. If you train in the morning, this should be your breakfast. Repeat this meal two hours later. These dosages are equivalent to 1.1 g/kg of carbs and 0.55 g/kg of protein. Your carbohydrate intake should be predominantly low glycemic-index carbs, although some simple sugars can be included. Count only proteins with a Biologic Value over 70 in your protein dosage unless you eat complementary proteins within a few hours.

If you train first thing in the morning and find that your energy level drops toward the end of your workout, part of the reason may be that you didn't eat enough carbs the night before. Try consuming the food that you used to eat before your workout during the previous evening. This will replenish your glycogen stores and should provide ample energy for your workout. Experiment with this technique, as it will produce the most beneficial hormone response from exercise.

Some athletes with high metabolisms may find, however, that they still feel sluggish without some nourishment before their morning workout. If this happens to you, drink a half-cup of juice and 25 g of whey protein as soon as you get up (even before showering and drinking coffee). This modest intake of simple sugars and easily digestible protein will pass quickly through your digestive tract, allowing your blood-sugar level to return to normal by the time you actually start your workout. Do not exceed these quantities or switch to complex carbs or solid protein sources, however, as this will slow digestion and produce counterproductive changes in hormone levels.

Regardless of when you train, never skip breakfast. It truly is one of the most important meals of the day, giving you the opportunity to supply your body with the nutrients it needs after a sleep-time fast of at least eight hours. Also, if you are fond of nutrition/energy bars or drinks, consume them after your workout. You'll get a greater hormonal response and better results from your training program.

28.

CONSUME A VARIETY OF FOODS

Eating the same thing every day gets boring. It's also not healthy. Each protein source has a somewhat different combination of amino acids. By varying the types of protein you eat, you provide the broadest spectrum of these vital nutrients for muscle growth. Vegetables and fruits also have different vitamin and mineral profiles. A variety of foods will help ensure a well-balanced diet and could even boost your testosterone level.

Athletes are creatures of habit. Once they develop a diet that works, they often stick with it for extended periods. This can make preparation easier because you can cook up large batches of baked chicken breasts and other favorites at once. It can also provide a stable intake of calories as long as your daily portions remain constant. However, eating the same foods all of the time can actually hurt your progress. You need to include a variety of different proteins and carbohydrates in your diet program.

Each protein source has its own unique blend of amino acids.

Even complete proteins contain variations in their amino acid compositions, which is part of the reason why proteins have different Biologic Values. (For a chart of Biologic Values, see page 79.) Yet, you can't rely solely on Biologic Value to determine your protein selections. Whey, for example, has a value of 104 but has less glutamine and arginine than casein or soy with their values in the 70s. (Only essential amino acids are included in the calculations of Biologic Value.) In order to ensure a full spectrum of all of the amino acids, you need to eat a variety of different foods, including chicken, turkey, fish, dairy products, soy, and even lean beef or pork occasionally. Select protein sources with a low fat content, of course, but make it a point to vary what you eat.

The same principle applies to vegetables and other carbohydrates. Each source of carbohydrates has its own unique blend of nutrients, including essential vitamins and minerals. Fiber content also varies among the edible parts of plants. Although starchy carbs such as pasta, potato, rice, and grains have lower nutrient profiles than vegetables, even these carbohydrates should be alternated in your diet program.

Another way to add variation to your diet is to use seasonings. Spices and herbs are full of flavor, but have no calories. They titillate your taste buds and make your meals something special. With a change in seasoning, you can create a delicious meal in a few minutes that will be a welcome break from eating the same thing all of the time.

There's more to meal variety than just keeping your mind interested in eating. It can actually impact your hormone levels. Sometimes athletes eat a diet consisting largely of protein. A study by Anderson compared the hormonal response of a high-protein diet (44 percent of total calories) with a diet that contained a moderate level of protein and more carbohydrates (70 percent of the total). The high-carbohydrate diet produced a higher level of testosterone and a lower level of cortisol than this high-protein diet. So when you provide your body with a variety of carbohydrates and limit your protein consumption to the levels that are recommended in this book, you not only get more nutritious and enjoyable meals, you could also boost your supply of a major anabolic hormone while reducing the quantity of a catabolic hormone. Yet another reason to make variety a founding principle of your diet program.

29.

DRINK PLENTY
OF WATER

Water is an essential yet frequently overlooked nutrient. Your muscles are up to 70-percent water, and adequate hydration is essential for muscle function and growth. In fact, protein synthesis is increased when the muscles are fully hydrated. Eat plenty of foods with high water content, and drink $1\frac{1}{2}$ to 2 liters of water each day (about six to eight glasses). This is particularly important in summer when you lose significant amounts of water due to sweating.

Water is very important for the athlete. While you can live with deficiencies of most nutrients for days or even weeks, a few days without water will kill you. There is more water in the body than any other nutrient. Up to 60 percent of a person's total body weight is water. It comprises up to 70 percent of the weight of muscle but only 25 percent of the weight of fat.

Water plays a role in digestion, assimilation, circulation and excretion. It is the major ingredient in blood plasma, which transports nutrients and gases between the cells. It is also a necessary part of many chemical reactions in the body. Water carries off the waste products of energy metabolism from the cell and provides the fluid needed to get rid of the body's wastes. These wastes include the urea that is produced during the breakdown of dietary protein. Water also lubricates the joints and gives form to the muscles.

The body produces a significant amount of water when food molecules are broken down for energy. In fact, nearly 25 percent of the total daily water requirement for a sedentary person can be provided by this metabolic mechanism. Each gram of glucose combines with 2.7 g of water to form glycogen in the muscles and liver. This water is released when the glycogen is converted into energy.

One of the most important functions of water is heat regulation. Exercise generates heat, which can severely impact the functioning of the body if the temperature rises too high. When water is released through the skin and evaporates, heat is dissipated into the environment, lowering the skin temperature. This air-conditioning function can use up a great deal of water depending on the intensity and duration of exercise and the environmental conditions of relative humidity and air temperature. While a limited amount of water can be lost without affecting sports performance (up to 2 percent of body weight), a loss of only 3 percent can reduce endurance. Even greater losses can impact muscular strength. When the water loss exceeds 6 percent of bodyweight, life-threatening symptoms such as heat exhaustion and heat stroke can occur.

Dehydration causes the blood volume to go down, forcing the heart to work harder. It also interferes with numerous body functions, including protein synthesis in muscle. Dehydration can actually be speeded up by high-protein diets, since water is diverted to the kidneys to get rid of the excess urea produced by these diets. One way to avoid dehydration is to keep protein intake moderate while consuming water at regular intervals throughout your training sessions. This is especially important in hot weather and during endurance activities like long-distance marathons.

Make sure you get enough water every day, particularly during workouts. Eat plenty of fruits and vegetables that are high in water content, and drink $1\frac{1}{2}$ to 2 liters of water each day (about six to eight glasses). While weight training, have a few sips of water between sets, even if you're not thirsty. Thirst is not a very sensitive indicator of water need.

Avoid sugary sodas and other sucrose-based drinks, including those fruit-juice blends that are only partially juice. Sports drinks made from glucose polymers and fructose are better, but natural fruit juices are best. However, juices have no fiber and are relatively high in calories, so they should only make up a small portion of the diet, especially when you are on a reduced-calorie diet to lower your bodyweight. In these situations your body would rather feel the sensation of fullness that comes from solid food. You're better off eating the fruit with its greater nutrient value than the juice made from it. In fact, the best thing to drink is plain water.

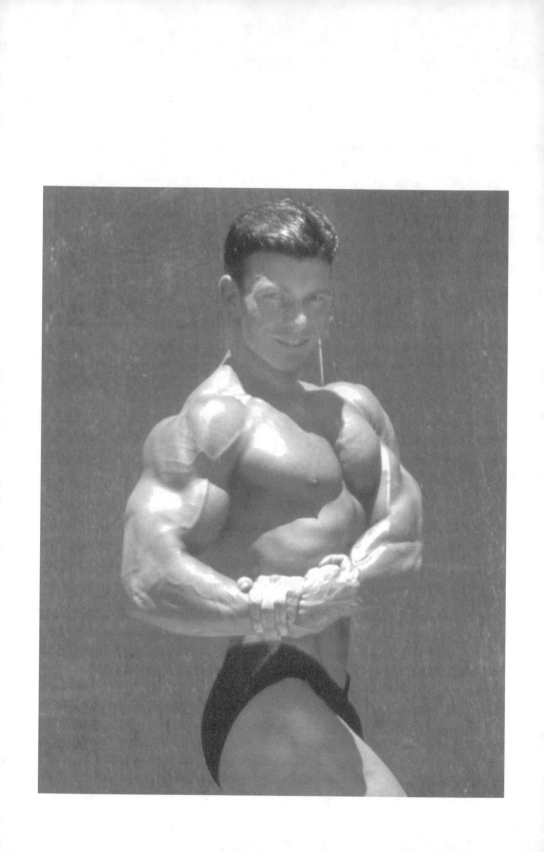

30.

STAY RELATIVELY LEAN ALL YEAR

Yo-yo dieting destroys muscle tissue. In order to achieve the greatest long-term gains, you need to stay relatively lean all year. You don't want to starve yourself, but you shouldn't overeat either. A controlled food intake with adequate quantities of protein, carbohydrates, and fats will allow your body to build permanent muscle mass without generating the body fat that can hide your hard-earned gains.

Athletes want to build muscle as quickly as possible. Sometimes they try to achieve this by eating large amounts of food to increase their bodyweight. The rationale behind this practice is that heavier athletes tend to lift more weight. This additional weight, it is felt, will lead to more stimulation of the muscle fibers and consequent growth. Unfortunately, this thinking confuses muscle weight with total bodyweight. Clearly, athletes with more muscle mass will be able to lift more. However, body fat (adipose tissue) is not involved in muscle contraction. Simply put, adding a tire around your waist will not bring you the gains you seek.

Too much carbohydrate, fat, or even protein results in bodyfat deposition. This is a fact of life. Your body needs only so much of each nutrient every day. While the correct amount depends on your muscle mass, basal metabolic rate, and exercise intensity, every athlete has his or her own nutritional requirements. Bringing your diet up to these levels will enhance muscle growth. Anything beyond that point is diverted to the bodyfat stores.

Adipose tissue is nothing more than energy storage. One pound of bodyfat contains approximately 3,500 calories. Due to the nature of progressive resistance training, the recruitment of these fat stores during an exercise is minimal. While moderate-intensity exercise such as aerobics can utilize adipose tissue for fuel, the body is also capable of metabolizing carbohydrates for energy. There is simply no reason to carry around muscle-obscuring fat deposits under the pretext of improving your strength or performance. In fact, in any sport where speed is involved, these fat stores will slow you down.

While it is true that bodyfat provides resistance during squats and a few other exercises, you can achieve the same results by adding a plate to each side of the bar. And there are very few exercises where the entire body is in motion in this manner. Extra girth around your waist will not improve your biceps curl or bench press, for example.

Research has shown that yo-yo dieting is unhealthy. Bodyweight cycling can result in higher blood pressure and has been correlated with the risk of cardiovascular disease. The body also shows a higher preference for dietary fat once the athlete goes off the diet's restrictions. So staying relatively lean all year is not just a matter of looking good—your long-term health and quality of life can be impacted when you abuse your body with yo-yo dieting.

Try to listen to your body's requests for food and not your mind's desires. Eat when you are hungry, but only until you begin to feel full. Enjoy the good, healthy food you consume, for it is the raw material producing the muscle mass you desire. But don't shovel down food thinking that you are somehow building extra muscle in the process. With appropriate food consumption, you will create the maximum muscle growth with a minimum of bodyfat. The positive feedback you get when people see your defined physique will also inspire greater confidence in your abilities, leading to heavier lifts. The enjoyable result will be greater size gains.

31.

SPLURGE EVERY ONCE IN A WHILE

An excessively strict diet can reduce your motivation over time. While you need to watch what you eat in order to provide nutritional support for your muscle growth, this doesn't mean that your diet has to be tedious and unfulfilling. Enjoy an occasional splurge. Just keep the amount of the splurge moderate so you don't gain bodyfat. If there isn't enough protein in your splurge meal, have a protein shake or can of tuna when you get home.

Committed athletes want to do everything they can to build muscle and improve performance. They are disciplined, and recognize that a small hardship today is an acceptable price to pay for the greater sports benefits they will achieve in the long run. It is this sense of direction and vision that inspires us to train hard and watch what we eat. Yet, it can sometimes lead us to pursue diets that are excessively strict or even unhealthy. Once an athlete has decided on a nutritional program, he or she may rigidly follow it to the exclusion of all else. Most of the time, this single-mindedness is good. Other times it can be overkill, resulting in diminished drive and motivation.

Of course, athletic greatness is not achieved with a daily diet of pizza, ice cream, and French fries. On the other hand, you don't need to restrict yourself to foods that only a rabbit would love. You can have an occasional splurge without feeling guilty. Just try to keep the number of splurges fairly low.

Some athletes consider Sunday their splurge day. On this special day, they eat foods that would normally not be on their list. And as long as this splurge occurs only once a week, there is nothing wrong with it—provided that the amount of food eaten is not excessive. Now, there is nothing magical about Sunday. Any day will do. You could even have mini-splurges a couple of times per week, savoring the taste of a special treat without gorging yourself on it. The most important thing to remember is portion control. If you are going out with friends and they order pizza, you can have a slice. You could even have a frozen dessert. But there is no law that says you have to finish that pint of ice cream just because you started it! As long as you watch the total number of calories and the nutrients you consume each day, you will be able to enjoy an occasional splurge.

While splurging, getting enough carbohydrates and fat is rarely a problem. Yet, protein can be. If you are eating at a restaurant with small meat portions, don't panic. Enjoy your splurge. When you get home, have a protein shake or a can of tuna to ensure adequate amino-acid supplies. And if your splurge was a bit over the top, try to cut back on your calorie consumption the next day. When it comes to splurges, a bit of discipline and common sense goes a long way. Let reason be your guide. It will make your diet a lot more interesting, and will ensure that you stick with your predominantly healthy nutrition program over the long term.

32.

MAKE SURE YOU GET ENOUGH VITAMINS AND MINERALS

Vitamins and minerals are essential for good health and peak performance. Athletes have higher requirements for these micronutrients than sedentary individuals. Even though most athletes eat relatively large quantities of nutritious food, supplementation is often still necessary. You should take a multi-vitamin and multi-mineral tablet/capsule that provides 100 percent of the RDA twice per day. Additional amounts of calcium, magnesium, and the antioxidant vitamins C and E are also recommended.

Athletes need to be sure they consume sufficient vitamins and minerals. These micronutrients play vital roles in muscle development, energy production and many other essential functions. While they are often taken for granted, vitamins and minerals enable you to perform at your peak. Your micronutrient requirements go up as the intensity of your training increases, so you want to be sure you get enough. At the same time, taking more than you need will not provide an additional benefit. There are a number of excellent books that discuss vitamins and minerals at length, including *The Real Vitamin and Mineral Book* by Shari Leiberman and Nancy Bruning (Avery Publishing, 1998). Here are some basic facts to keep in mind.

There are currently thirteen vitamins that are recognized as essential for humans: vitamin A (retinol), B_1 (thiamine), B_2 (riboflavin), B_3 (niacin), B_6 (pyridoxine), B_{12} (cobalamin), pantothenic acid, folic acid, biotin, C, D, E and K. Even though your body's requirements for these nutrients are small compared with the macronutrients, a deficiency of any one of them can lead to illness and disease.

Vitamins are required for many different chemical reactions within the body. They help regulate the chain of metabolic reactions that controls tissue synthesis and the release of energy in food. Vitamin B_1, for example, plays a significant role in energy production. Without the right vitamins, these chemical reactions cannot take place at the proper rates, impacting the body's metabolic processes. Some vitamins also act as antioxidants, protecting the body from potentially cancer-causing compounds called free radicals.

There are two types of vitamins: fat-soluble and water-soluble. The fat-soluble vitamins (A, D, E, and K) can only be dissolved in fat. A small amount of fat must therefore be included in the diet so that these vitamins can be assimilated and used by the body. Fat-soluble vitamins that are not immediately needed are stored in the adipose tissues for later use, so deficiencies of this type of vitamins are relatively rare. In fact, because these vitamins remain in the system for so long, athletes who take extremely high levels of fat-soluble vitamins can actually develop toxic levels in their bodies. For this reason, care should be taken when consuming fat-soluble vitamin supplements.

The water-soluble vitamins (B-complex vitamins and vitamin C) act as coenzymes. They combine with other small protein molecules to form active enzymes. These vitamins dissolve in water but not in fat. As a result, they cannot be stored to any great degree by the body. Water-soluble vitamin supplies that are not immediately needed are likely to be excreted in the urine. It is therefore necessary to eat foods that contain these vitamins on a regular basis to prevent deficiencies.

Minerals are also essential for good health. Minerals are found in the body's enzymes and hormones, as well as in the structural elements of the body. While vitamins are able to facilitate chemical reactions in the body without actually becoming part of them, minerals usually become incorporated within the body's physical and chemical structures. They play an essential role in formation of the teeth and bones, and are involved in functions as diverse as maintaining a normal heartbeat and regulating the acid-base balance of the body. Minerals allow the muscles to contract and permit the nerves to transmit impulses. They also regulate cellular metabolism and stimulate various reactions that allow energy to be released from the foods we eat.

There are twenty-two minerals that are currently recognized as essential to human health: calcium, phosphorus, sulfur, potassium, chloride, sodium, magnesium, iron, fluorine, zinc, copper, selenium, iodine, chromium, cobalt, silicon, vanadium, tin, nickel, manganese, molybdenum, and lead. Minerals have been divided into two groups, known as major minerals and trace minerals, depending on the quantities of the mineral that are required for health. Individual minerals also vary in the degree to which they are absorbed by the body. This variation, called bioavailability, can range from as low as 5 percent for manganese to 30 to 40 percent for calcium and magnesium. The bioavailability of a mineral is taken into consideration when the Recommended Dietary Allowance for that mineral is established. It should be noted that the levels of toxicity for minerals are much lower than they are for vitamins. This is because minerals are metals, so they should be treated with a great deal of respect. Taking too many minerals can definitely harm your health without giving you any performance benefit in return.

Athletes tend to eat relatively large quantities of good food. This dietary intake should provide a substantial portion of your total vitamin and mineral requirements. In some cases, it may supply all of an athlete's needs for a particular micronutrient. Also, bear in mind that vitamins have the ability to be used over and over in metabolic reactions, so there is not a direct correlation between activity levels and micronutrient needs. Still, many athletes will require additional vitamins and minerals to perform at their best. This can be achieved by taking a multi-vitamin/multi-mineral supplement that contains the Recommended Dietary Allowance for each micronutrient twice a day.

There are four micronutrients that are particularly important for muscular development: vitamin C, vitamin E, calcium, and magnesium. Several studies have shown sports benefits from these nutrients at levels significantly greater than the RDA, so you should take extra amounts of them in addition to your multi-vitamin/multi-mineral supplement.

Vitamin C is well known for its ability to help strengthen the immune system. This antioxidant vitamin can also help neutralize potentially damaging free radicals, which have been connected with a number of diseases. Vitamin C is involved in the formation of bone, teeth, and collagen. Researchers at the University of Cape Town, South Africa, gave 600 mg of the vitamin to participants of a 90-kilometer race. They found that supplementation significantly reduced the incidence of common cold symptoms during this acute physical stress, although not all studies have had this same result. Other placebo-controlled studies have shown that 1 to 2 g per day can decrease the severity of common cold symptoms. In order to keep your immune system in peak condition you should consume 1 to 2 g of vitamin C each day. Citrus fruits, tomatoes, green peppers, and green leafy vegetables contain good amounts of this vitamin. If you do not get enough from your diet, inexpensive tablets are available.

Vitamin E is another antioxidant vitamin. It is fat-soluble and is found primarily in cell membranes. Vitamin E helps prevent the free-radical damage that contributes to cardiovascular disease. It protects the red blood cells as well, and plays an essential role in cellular respiration in cardiac and skeletal muscle, which increases endurance and stamina.

Vitamin E also reduces the membrane disruption that occurs in exercised muscles due to increased free-radical production. A placebo-controlled study by McBride gave 1,200 IU of vitamin E to six weight-trained males for two weeks. The men were then asked to perform a vigorous whole-body workout after a two-day rest period. Vitamin E supplementation significantly reduced the muscle damage created by this workout program. You should consume 600 to 1,200 IU of vitamin E per day. Good food sources include grains, green leafy vegetables and seeds. Many oils contain vitamin E as well, but you may prefer to take a supplement to keep your calorie count down.

Vitamin E also appears to be necessary for the optimal uptake of creatine into muscle cells. A study by Gerber found that vitamin E deficiencies reduce creatine levels in the skeletal muscle of rats. Although such deficiencies are rare, this is one more reason to get enough vitamin E.

Calcium is the most abundant mineral in the human body. It assists in regulating the heartbeat and helps to build and maintain the bones and teeth. Calcium helps reduce lactic acid concentrations in the blood during and after exercise. It is also essential for muscle contraction. When a muscle fiber is stimulated to contract, calcium binds to one of the protein-based filaments deep inside the muscle cell, and, in effect, turns it on. When the nerve impulse to the muscle fiber is removed, the calcium ions move back to their storage location, which stops the contraction of the muscle. In order to ensure an adequate calcium supply, you should consume 10 mg of calcium per pound of bodyweight (25 mg/kg). Good food sources of calcium include nonfat milk and yogurt, mozzarella cheese, broccoli, and green leafy vegetables. If you don't get enough from your diet, you should buy calcium carbonate or calcium citrate tablets to make up the difference. These forms of calcium is more bioavailable than the less expensive bone-meal or oyster-shell products.

Magnesium helps control carbohydrate synthesis and is an essential activator of many enzyme systems. It counteracts the stimulatory effect of calcium in the muscle fibers and helps to prevent muscle cramps. A study by Lukaski at the University of North Dakota found that magnesium also enhances oxygen delivery to working muscles in trained subjects, while a study by Porta discovered that magnesium supplementation reduced the level of the catabolic hormone, cortisol. Despite its importance, the body contains less than an ounce (20 to 28 g) of magnesium, 27 percent of which is found in muscle. You should consume 3.5 mg of magnesium per pound of bodyweight (8 mg/kg). There are not many good food sources of magnesium except for cod, snapper, and some other seafoods. Whole grains and vegetables contain small amounts. Fortunately, magnesium tablets are inexpensive, so be sure you get an adequate supply of this essential mineral.

By providing your body with a balanced spectrum of micro-nutrients, you ensure that no vitamin or mineral becomes a limiting factor in your muscle growth. Given the moderate expense involved, you should make sure you get enough vitamins and minerals every day.

33.

USE CREATINE

Creatine is the most effective sports supplement currently available without a prescription. It is naturally produced by the body and plays an essential role in muscle contraction. Creatine supplementation has been shown to boost strength and power in scientific studies. It builds lean muscle mass by increasing the volume of the muscle cells and may also stimulate more protein synthesis. Take 4 to 12 grams of creatine per day (1 to 3 level teaspoons), depending on your exercise intensity and muscle mass. Divide this daily amount into two or three doses.

While scientists have known about creatine since the nineteenth century, it has only been available as a supplement since the early 1990s. Within a few short years, creatine skyrocketed in popularity to become the best-selling sports supplement ever. This natural compound is technically an amino acid. A small amount is produced in your body every day in the liver, pancreas, and kidneys from the amino acids arginine, glycine, and methionine. Small amounts of creatine are found in many body tissues, including the heart, brain, and testes. However, 95 percent of your creatine supply is in the skeletal muscles. There it plays an important role in muscular contraction, particularly during the explosive movements that are required for a number of sports.

More than fifty published studies have explored creatine's benefits. However, there is only enough space here to mention a few. (For more information on this supplement, read *Creatine: Nature's Muscle Builder*, Avery Publishing, 1997). Creatine increases your muscles' ability to perform physical work by permitting an essential energy-producing compound known as ATP to be resynthesized at a greater rate. By providing more fuel for continued muscle contraction, creatine lets you work out longer and more intensely. And the more work you do (whether it's lifting weights or swimming 100-meter sprints), the stronger you become over time. Creatine supplementation also reduces the muscles' dependence on the energy pathway that burns glucose and glycogen, which leads to less lactic acid production. This permits your muscles to work for a longer period of time before fatiguing. Over time, the increased work effort stimulates the body to produce additional muscle proteins as a training adaptation, resulting in enhanced strength and power.

Soon after you begin using creatine, you will feel your muscles getting larger and harder. This is due to an increase in the quantity of fluid stored inside your muscle cells. As the amount of this intracellular fluid rises, it pushes against the cell membrane and actually expands the cell's volume. The microscopic boost in mass, multiplied by the millions of muscle cells, results in bigger muscles. This process is technically known as volumization.

The increase in intracellular fluid levels is also thought to stimulate the synthesis of new muscle proteins, although the definitive research study on this topic has still not been completed. Studies by Haussinger and Waldegger show that an increase in cellular hydration acts as an anabolic signal in cells, which promotes protein synthesis. Scientists feel that creatine may also promote the uptake of amino acids into the cell. This could produce an increase in the quantity and thickness of two protein-based myofilaments known as actin and myosin, resulting in greater muscle mass over time.

Many people note improvements from creatine supplementation during their first week of use. "One of the most prominent benefits is the change in your body's ability to perform intense exercise," notes creatine pioneer Anthony Almada, MSc, currently an Adjunct Researcher at the University of Memphis in Tennessee. "There is a change in the way your body looks and feels. Your muscles feel harder and your clothing fits differently. There is also an increase in strength and fat-free mass as well as a possible reduction in body fat over time."

Several researchers have confirmed that creatine boosts lean mass, muscular strength and power. A 1995 study by Earnest and associates at Texas Women's University, University of Texas Southwestern Medical Center, and The Cooper Clinic in Dallas, Texas, gave eight weight-trained men 20 g of creatine per day for 28 days. The researchers discovered that there was a 3.7-lb (1.7-kg) increase in total body weight with only a 0.2-lb (0.1-kg) increase in body fat. This was a 2 percent gain in the athletes' average lean mass within 30 days. The average weight that the test subjects could lift on a set of bench presses with one repetition (1RM) rose by 8 kilograms, a gain of over 18 pounds. That's a 7 percent improvement in one month. The average number of repetitions the participants could lift at a weight that was only 70 percent of the 1RM also rose, from eleven to fifteen. The end result was that total lifting volume increased by 43 percent in only one month.

A 1997 study by Volek from the Center for Sports Medicine at Pennsylvania State University confirmed these results. After test subjects took 25 grams of creatine per day for a week, they experienced a significant improvement in peak power output during five sets of jump squats, along with a significant increase in the number of repetitions they could do during five sets of bench presses. They also gained an average of 3 pounds (1.4 kg) of body mass during the experiment. Additional studies on creatine have shown benefits for bodybuilders, powerlifters, and rowers. Depending on the event and the time between bouts, swimmers and track and field athletes can also benefit. Wrestlers, boxers, and baseball and football players would appear to benefit from the increases in strength, but no studies have yet determined the specific performance improvements in these sports.

With clinical studies such as these, it is no wonder that creatine has become as popular as it is. However, a few cautions are in order. First, not everyone responds to creatine supplementation. For unknown reasons, 20 to 30 percent of athletes do not benefit from creatine use. This may be due to the supply of creatine in their muscles before they started supplementing, but it could relate to other factors. Second, creatine can cause certain side effects, particularly if you take too much at once. "While virtually no side effects have been noticed in the studies on creatine, my clinical experience has been that creatine can cause nausea, diarrhea or stomach upset in some users, usually on dosages above 5 grams," notes Ray Sahelian, MD, co-author of *Creatine: Nature's Muscle Builder.* "If you get a side effect, you should reduce the size of each dose. This eliminates the problem in most instances." Third, while creatine appears to be exceptionally benign, there are no long-term studies yet on its use. You may wish to cycle your creatine supplementation to give your body a chance to produce creatine on its own every once in a while. (Supplementation appears to down-regulate the body's own creatine production.) Fourth, if you are having tests for kidney function, be sure to inform your physician about your creatine use. He or she could otherwise misinterpret the higher levels of a harmless by-product called creatinine and erroneously conclude that you have a kidney problem.

Creatine is usually sold as creatine monohydrate, which is a virtually tasteless white powder. It comes in two grain sizes: the traditional sugar-sized grain and a newer micronized version. Both are chemically the same. A new patented form of creatine, creatine citrate, is also available. Scientists know that it is assimilated into the bloodstream as effectively as creatine monohydrate, but no research has yet been published on its sports benefits. Liquid creatine contains creatine monohydrate in solution. There is considerable debate on the stability of the product, however. Until this situation is clarified, you may wish to avoid using liquid creatine.

You should take 4 to 12 grams (1 to 3 level teaspoons) of creatine per day divided into two to three doses. One of these daily doses should be taken after your workout to help replenish the amount metabolized during exercise. The ideal dosage depends on your muscle mass and exercise intensity. The more muscle you have, the more creatine you need. However, if you consume too much, the excess will be excreted in your urine. Experiment with your creatine supplementation to see what dosage works best for you.

A study by Green found that creatine concentrations in muscle rose an additional 36 percent on average when the study participants added nearly 100 grams of simple sugars to the 5 grams of creatine they consumed. This is because the sugars stimulated an insulin response, which helped to transport creatine into the muscle cells. However, 100 grams is quite a load of sugar, and it may not be healthy to consume this amount on a regular basis. Anecdotal evidence suggests that smaller amounts of carbohydrates are also effective. Fruit and vegetable juices are good options as creatine vehicles. Juices contain large amounts of fructose and other simple sugars. They also contain significant amounts of vitamins, minerals, carotenoids, and flavonoids, which have health benefits. A number of supplement companies also sell creatine/carbohydrate products that are effective. Don't take your creatine with caffeinated beverages, however. A study by Vandenberghe discovered that the equivalent of five cups of coffee eliminated creatine's performance benefits in the short term.

Creatine can be taken with meals when you find it more convenient to do so. Although the fat and protein in the meal may reduce the insulin response achieved, the creatine is apparently still absorbed by the muscle cells as long as the meal contains sufficient carbohydrates, such as a baked potato, bread, rice or pasta. You could also take your creatine with a protein shake as long as there are carbohydrates in the shake or you eat carbs at the same time. Mixing creatine with food would minimize any gastrointestinal discomfort and is a preferred option for people with sensitive stomachs.

While not everyone benefits from creatine use, most people get favorable results. Creatine is fairly inexpensive as supplements go, so give it a try. You may well find that it boosts your strength and muscle mass in a quick, visible way.

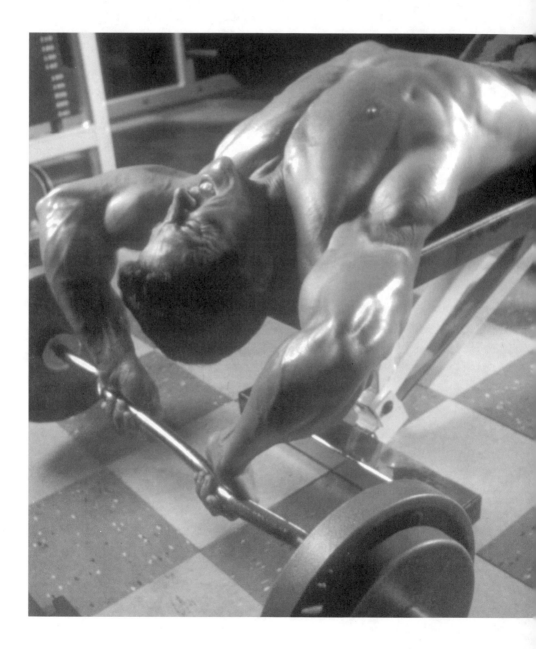

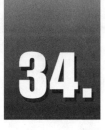

34.

TAKE GLUTAMINE

Glutamine is an amino acid that plays many vital roles in the body. It reduces the build-up of lactic acid due to exercise and increases the production of growth hormone, permitting more effective training sessions. Glutamine also helps regulate protein synthesis and improves immune system function. Take 5 grams of glutamine (1 rounded teaspoon) before your workout. Consume 2 to 3 grams on an empty stomach several times a day to maximize your growth-hormone secretion.

During the past few years, there has been a wealth of new information published in scientific journals about glutamine. Previously, it had been felt that the body could always produce a sufficient quantity of this amino acid on its own. This was the reasoning behind the traditional classification of glutamine as a nonessential amino acid. Research has now shown that this is not the case for many athletes. Due to their increased activity levels and metabolic requirements, athletes can develop deficiencies of glutamine that may hold them back in their training progress. In these situations, glutamine supplementation can remove a limiting factor and help the athlete to achieve his or her optimal performance.

Glutamine is the most abundant amino acid in the human body. The majority of this glutamine is stored within the skeletal muscles, although significant amounts are also found in the blood, lungs, liver, and brain. Because it has a nitrogen atom to spare, glutamine is able to transport nitrogen around the body. This "shuttle" activity helps it to neutralize the lactic acid that builds up during exercise. The greater the availability of glutamine, the greater the potential for rapid restoration of the body's acid-base balance. This can allow exercise to resume sooner and may even permit higher levels of force production during your workout.

Glutamine also acts as a nitrogen precursor for several coenzymes and the phosphate molecules that muscles use for energy production. In addition, glutamine provides fuel for the mucosal cells of the intestinal wall, which helps to promote the maximum assimilation of vital nutrients for athletic activity. It also plays a role in the maintenance of protein balance in muscle by increasing protein synthesis and reducing protein breakdown. The more glutamine in the muscle cells, the higher the rate of protein synthesis. This is because glutamine increases the amount of fluid inside the muscle cell, which is a powerful, anabolic signal for the building of new proteins. Glutamine supplementation has even been shown to reduce the muscle wasting associated with high cortisol levels.

Glutamine can increase the production of growth hormone (hGH). Secreted by the pituitary gland, hGH has a major role in muscle growth and retention due to its ability to promote cell division and proliferation throughout the body. It does this by increasing the amount of amino acids transported inside the cell membrane, which provides raw material for the synthesis of additional proteins in the muscle fiber. Growth hormone promotes the growth of the bones and connective tissues as well, including cartilage, tendons, and ligaments. It even increases the level of free fatty acids in the blood, resulting in greater use of fats as an energy source and the sparing of available proteins and carbohydrates. By raising the body's energy expenditure at rest, hGH helps to reduce your body-fat level, too.

A recent study by Welbourne found that oral glutamine supplementation has a dramatic impact on growth hormone secretion.

Nine healthy volunteers aged 32 to 64 consumed 2 g of glutamine over a 20-minute period that started 45 minutes after a light breakfast. During the next 90 minutes, blood samples were obtained every half-hour and measured for hGH and bicarbonate levels. The researchers found that growth hormone levels rose 430 percent over baseline levels after 90 minutes. There was a dramatic rise in plasma bicarbonate concentration as well.

Strenuous exercise taxes the immune system. There is a higher incidence of infections and cold symptoms after a bout of intense exercise. A study by Castell found that there is a decrease in the plasma level of glutamine in endurance athletes after a marathon. This reduction continues for one hour, then slowly returns to normal sixteen hours after the event. During this period there is also a drop in the number of lymphocytes (white blood cells), which are dependent on glutamine for optimal growth. The decline in lymphocyte count, along with other negative changes in the immune system, are considered by many researchers to be the cause of the increased frequency of illness among athletes.

Here again, glutamine can help. Another study by Castell found a correlation between oral glutamine consumption and the absence of illness in trained athletes. He measured the levels of infection in more than 200 runners and rowers. Middle-distance runners had the lowest infection rate, while the rowers and full- or ultra-marathon runners had the highest levels. Castell then gave a total of 5 g of glutamine to half of these athletes while the others drank a placebo. Half of the dosage was taken right after the exercise bout and the remainder was consumed two hours after exercise. The results were dramatic. Only 19 percent of the athletes using glutamine reported infections during the next seven days, while 51 percent of the athletes on the placebo came down with a cold or similar infection. Given how frustrated athletes get when they are forced to take time off, supplementation with glutamine would seem to be great health insurance.

Even though the body produces 50 to 120 grams of glutamine on its own each day, supplementation has been shown to provide additional benefits. While part of your dose winds up being metabolized by the mucosal cells of the small intestine, it is still beneficial because the body uses this source instead of getting the glutamine it needs from your muscles. You can minimize this drain on your muscle stores by taking 5 g of glutamine right before your workouts. This will help to reduce lactic-acid concentrations during exercise as well.

You should also consume 2 to 3 g of glutamine with a glass of water several times per day to stimulate hGH secretion. Tomas Welbourne, author of the study that discovered the glutamine/hGH connection, notes that high blood-sugar levels prevent glutamine from promoting hGH release, so be sure to take it at least one hour after a meal and one hour before your next one. Stick to the recommended dosage, however, as greater amounts can cause the liver to degrade the glutamine before it gets to the pituitary gland to do its job. Once again, more is not necessarily better.

Bear in mind that glutamine is not creatine, so you won't feel anything happening. Still, the research on this amino acid is very encouraging. Add it to your supplementation program and see how it can help you stay healthy and strong.

35.

TRY MSM

MSM has been around for decades, but only recently have athletes discovered its benefits for training. It can dramatically reduce the delayed-onset muscle soreness that occurs with intense exercise. Start with a dose of 2 grams and slowly increase the dosage to 5 grams over several weeks. Take two doses on training days (one before your workout and another afterward). One dose is sufficient on rest days. MSM crystals have a bitter taste, so you will probably want to use capsules.

Athletes who push it to the limit with their weight training frequently experience delayed-onset muscle soreness. This soreness is caused by the microcellular damage that can occur from the stresses of your training program. At the microscopic level, the protein myofilaments that permit muscle contraction lose some of their structural integrity. Other parts of the muscle fiber can also be damaged. Some scientists speculate that the lactic acid produced during your sets irritates these injured tissues as well, further increasing the damage. The soreness can begin within hours and often continues for several days after your workout.

MSM supplementation can dramatically reduce this muscle soreness. This white, crystalline powder, technically known as methylsulfonylmethane, is effective in reducing inflammation. It also inhibits pain impulses along nerve fibers. MSM dilates blood vessels and increases blood flow as well, which could help to reduce the amount of irritating lactic acid inside the muscle cell. However, its mechanism(s) of action remain a mystery at this time.

It is widely assumed that MSM works because it is a bioavailable source of sulfur. (One-third of the MSM molecule is sulfur by weight.) Sulfur is found in virtually all tissues, particularly the red blood cells, muscle, skin, hair, and nails. It is involved in a number of endocrine and neurotransmitter functions. Sulfur also provides raw material for many enzymes and for compounds that protect against toxicity and free-radical damage. Sulfur is the eighth most abundant element in the human body, comprising 0.25 to 0.5 percent of your body weight. Despite these facts, there is no RDA for this vital mineral.

Sulfur is contained in four amino acids: the essential amino acid methionine and the nonessential cysteine, cystine, and taurine. Nutritionists have historically assumed that if you eat enough protein, you will get enough sulfur. However, these are the same people who think that you don't have to take vitamins if you eat right. While this may be true for a couch potato, it is certainly not true for an athlete. So you may still have a sulfur deficiency that is holding back your gains, even though you eat more protein than the average person does. It should be noted, however, that there has been little research into sulfur deficiencies, so this is merely a hypothesis as to why MSM works.

Many athletes report that their soreness drops by as much as 40 percent when they take MSM. Some note that they don't have to use the railing any more to climb stairs the day after their leg workout! Even better, the decrease in microcellular damage lessens the amount of repair work needed inside the muscle fiber, giving the body more time to build new muscle tissue. Strength levels often increase, permitting more intense workouts. This can lead to greater muscle mass over time, provided of course that you eat right and don't overtrain.

"MSM helps to alleviate the inevitable muscle soreness that comes with peak-intensity training," notes Mike Torchia, a fitness consultant and overall winner at the 1977 Collegiate Mr. America. "It quickly relieves the soreness, so I can continue training hard." He has also found that it helps him to build muscle. "It's a no-brainer. Less muscle damage means that more of your body's efforts can go into packing on more mass. It's been a great help."

It seems clear that MSM can give your workouts a major boost. Unlike creatine and glutamine, however, which have been extensively studied, there is little published research so far on MSM. We do know that it is a metabolite of DMSO, a prescription drug that has been the subject of more than 15,000 studies over the past 45 years. (About 15 percent of the DMSO molecule metabolizes into MSM in the body.) Logically, if there were a problem with 15 percent of this molecule, it would have shown up by now. MSM also appears to be safe. In fact, a study performed at one of the world's leading toxicology centers in Italy found that it is less toxic than table salt. Still, there are big holes in our knowledge of MSM.

Your body contains tiny amounts of MSM naturally (about 2 parts per million). This comes from food sources such as milk, vegetables, coffee and tea. In order to get enough to help your workouts, however, you need to supplement. MSM comes in crystal form and in capsules. The crystals are much less expensive, but you may find the bitter taste to be intolerable. If you decide to try crystals, buy a small container. Drink it with juice or other strong-flavored liquid to mask the taste, and have a chaser of water ready. A level teaspoon of crystals contains 5 g of MSM. Capsules, of course, have no unpleasant taste, but they are more expensive. The decision is yours.

Begin your supplementation with a dose of 2 g. Some athletes who have taken too much too quickly have experienced headaches. It is better to give your body time to adjust to the higher MSM levels. After a week, increase the dosage to 3 g and then increase it to 4 and 5 g respectively over the next two weeks. Take one dose before your workout and another dose afterward. This will ensure the greatest concentration of MSM during your training session and the post-workout recovery phase. On the days that you don't work out, a single dose is sufficient. Taking it with meals will reduce the likelihood of any gastrointestinal upset. Also, some athletes say that it increases their energy level. If you notice this, don't take it before bedtime, as it may keep you awake. Other benign side effects include smoother skin and stronger nails.

Although MSM is usually quite safe, a few precautions are in order. Clinical observations indicate that it has an aspirin-like effect on platelet aggregation, which results in thinner blood. "If you are taking high doses of aspirin or other blood-thinning medications, consult with your physician before taking MSM," says Ronald Lawrence, MD, president of the American Medical Athletic Association and co-author of *The Miracle of MSM: The Natural Solution for Pain* (Putnam, 1999). "Also, MSM may interfere with the accuracy of a test for liver damage that measures enzyme levels, so inform your doctor if you are supplementing with this nutrient." In addition, approximately 1 percent of users may experience a rash, particularly in warmer climates. If this occurs, reducing the dosage will usually eliminate the problem.

The buzz about MSM gets stronger with each passing day. More and more athletes are discovering that it reduces the soreness they get from their workouts, even though the amount of weight they can lift actually goes up. This often leads to greater muscle growth and a new enthusiasm at the gym. So give MSM a try. It could eliminate a nutrient deficiency that has been holding back your training progress.

36.

TAILOR YOUR SUPPLEMENT PROGRAM TO YOUR SPECIFIC NEEDS AND BUDGET

Unless you're one of the fortunate few, your financial resources are limited. You may need to select from the various supplements available based on your budget and the specific needs of your sport. Protein, particularly whey protein, is a good place to start, followed by creatine and a vitamin/mineral supplement. You may also wish to experiment with glutamine and MSM if you can afford them. However, whole food should comprise most of your diet.

In a perfect world, we would all have the resources to buy whatever we wanted. Alas, the world is far from perfect. Many of us have real financial constraints that limit what we can purchase. We need to make choices between whole foods, supplements and other necessities like rent and utilities. In this situation, it is important to get the biggest bang for your buck. You need to make hard decisions based on the specific needs of your sport and the amount of cash you have available.

One of the best ways to stretch your dollar is to buy in bulk.

Supplements are no different than foods at the supermarket. The bigger the package, the less you pay per ounce. While it will set you back a bit paying for the larger size initially, in the long run you wind up saving money. This is particularly true for creatine and glutamine, although the same principle applies to most supplements. Also, buy powders instead of capsules. It is expensive to put powder into a gelatin capsule, and that cost is passed on to you. You often get at least twice as much of a supplement when you buy it in powder form, so save your change and spend it on something else.

Also, tailor your supplement and protein dosages to the requirements of your sport. You want to use the smallest amount of a supplement that works for you. By and large, sports that involve intense lifting or force production require higher nutrient levels than endurance-type sports. People with more muscle mass also need more nutrients than do athletes who are slimmer or shorter in stature. Another factor is your exercise intensity. Clearly, athletes who train long and hard need more supplements and protein than those who exercise less frequently and with lower intensity. Make an honest evaluation of your true requirements and only take as much as you really need. The rest is just wasted.

If you are on a budget, focus first on your protein requirements. Protein is an essential nutrient for muscle growth, and without adequate protein your muscles will not get larger even if all of the other nutrients are there in abundance. Whey protein is a particularly good source of the required amino acids, although some of the milk and egg and modified soy powders also provide high quality protein. Once you have made sure that you get enough protein, add creatine and a vitamin/mineral supplement to your list. Creatine is very inexpensive nowadays and it offers a lot of value for strength athletes. Vitamins and minerals are also essential for optimal growth, although true deficiencies are unlikely when you consume substantial amounts of good food. If you still have money left over, try glutamine and MSM. They promote a more anabolic environment for muscle growth and may help you in your quest to gain size.

However, you need to keep the whole issue of supplements in perspective. These products are intended to supplement your food intake, not substitute for it. While there are some excellent meal-replacement powders on the market, you should not live on them. Whole food has additional benefits. A well-selected variety of whole foods provides a full range of vitamins, minerals, flavonoids and other nutrients. Whole food also has fiber, which has important health benefits of its own. There is something to be said for having three square meals a day. The ideal role of these protein and meal-replacement powders is to provide a convenient way to get your fourth or fifth meals each day without the fat, cholesterol and excessive calories that two additional whole-food meals could provide. They are also more convenient, allowing you to eat good food on the run when you are in a hurry. They clearly have their place in a balanced diet, but they can be more expensive than whole food. If you're on a budget, use these and all supplements appropriately. Your wallet may start to bulge along with your muscles!

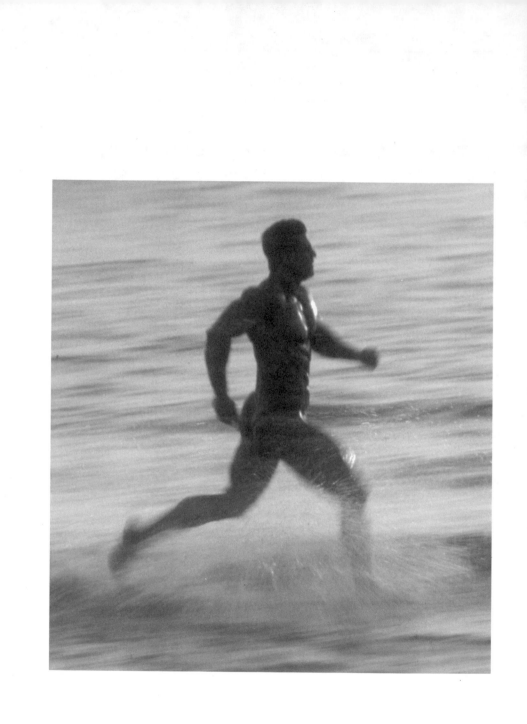

PART THREE

LIFESTYLE

INTRODUCTION

As an athlete, training is an important part of your life. You make sacrifices to achieve the muscle mass you seek. This involves a high-intensity exercise program that stimulates the muscle fibers to grow as well as a diet and supplementation program that provides your body with the nutrients it needs for maximum size gains. These are important variables in your overall strategy for growth. Yet, they are not sufficient in and of themselves.

Even the most well-designed exercise routine will not deliver the goods if you do not support it with an appropriate lifestyle. Nor will an impeccable diet and supplement regimen. In order to make permanent increases in strength and size, you have to integrate these variables into a larger whole.

You have probably heard about mind over matter. Well, there's such a thing as mind over muscle. The neural signals that govern muscle contraction originate in the brain, and if your brain is somewhat out of commission because you're hung over, stressed out or feeling down in the dumps, your training will suffer. It's as simple as that. In Part Three, fourteen of these lifestyle-related growth techniques are discussed. Together, they show how you can maximize your gains through modest lifestyle adjustments.

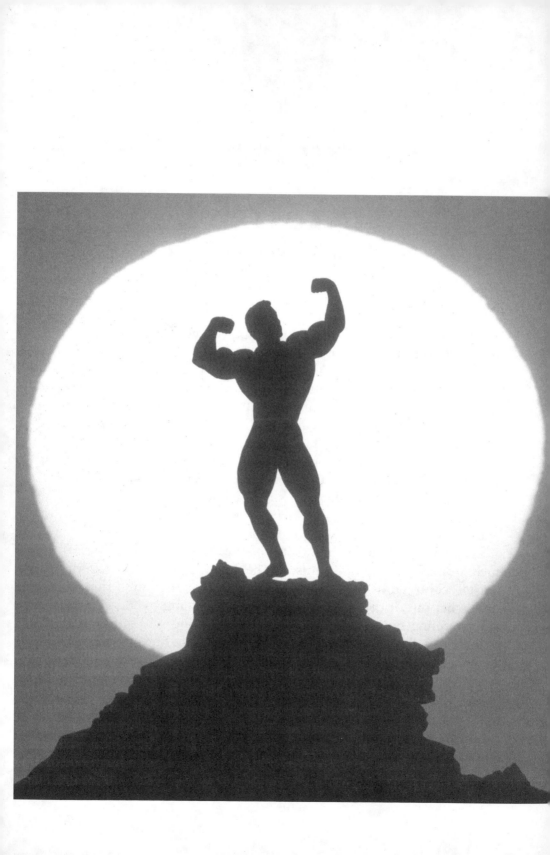

EXERCISE WHEN YOU ARE AT YOUR PEAK

Everyone has an internal clock that regulates his or her biological processes. Some people are "morning people," while others shine in the afternoon or evening. You should train when your energy level is at its peak. This will maximize your intensity and ensure the greatest possible gains.

At times you hear athletes and personal trainers insist on a specific time of day for a workout. Some people say that you can only make real gains when you train first thing in the morning, while others are just as adamant in support of afternoon or evening workouts. However, these one-size-fits-all approaches to training do not take into account our unique characteristics as individual athletes.

Everyone has their own biological clock, which regulates the body's activities during the course of the day. Some people happen to be morning people. They have a burst of energy during the first hours that the sun is around. These people can hop out of bed and hit the ground running, because they are entering what for them is the best part of the day. Arise and shine! Other equally devoted athletes feel that turning off the alarm clock is the first of many burdensome tasks that must be accomplished before their energy kicks in, something that may not occur until after lunch.

A biological clock isn't good or bad, any more than it is good or bad that the sun rises in the east. It is what it is. You simply have to adapt the pattern of your day's activities to your own biological clock and use it to your best advantage. You should train when your energy level is at its peak, because it is at this time of day (and only at this time) that you will be able to achieve maximum intensity and drive. You should go to the gym when you can create the highest amount of positive emotion for your workout, that is, at the time where your passion for training is at its peak. This will allow you to generate the greatest force to push or pull a weight against gravity. If you achieve these levels of intensity in the morning, that's when you should schedule your workouts. And if your feelings about packing on size reach their zenith in the afternoon or evening, this is when you need to make it to the gym.

It is, of course, possible that you will be at work when your energy level is at its peak. If your boss is a reasonable person, ask for a long lunch break or flexible work hours so you can accommodate the needs of your career and sport at the same time. If your work hours are more rigid, at least train when your energy level is as close to its peak as possible.

Work *with* your body, not against it. Despite the claims of some advocates, there is no "Universal Rule of Training Time." Once you get in tune with your biological clock and learn to sense its rhythms and fluctuations, you will be well on the way to achieving a sense of balance and oneness with your body. It will return the favor by giving you the quickest and largest gains in muscle mass.

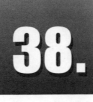

38.

TAKE A DISCIPLINED APPROACH

Discipline is a key part of your training program. Too much exercise will keep your body from recuperating and growing as rapidly as it otherwise could. Too little exercise or an undisciplined approach to your diet will also hold you back. By harnessing your knowledge and energy toward the fulfillment of your training goals, you can provide your body with the ideal amount of growth stimulation.

Discipline is essential to achieving your goals in sports and life in general. There are always plenty of distractions around and never enough time to do everything you want. Being disciplined helps you to sift through these difficult choices and establish priorities. This allows you to keep to the goals you have set without impulsive deviations that could take you off course. Once you have set a training schedule, you keep to it without skipping days. You follow your diet plan, recognizing that if you eat too much now you'll only have to over-diet later to make up for it. You choose your path and stick to it.

Discipline also gives you the stamina to persevere through bad times without giving up. There will inevitably be times that you reach sticking points in your training. A disciplined approach will keep you on track, helping you to overcome periods of moodiness or depression. A journey of a thousand miles, as any disciplined person will tell you, begins with a single step.

You need to integrate the various aspects of your life into a disciplined, rational system that will produce the results you seek. Kurt Elder, coach of the Gold's Gym Venice powerlifting team and the 1998 California state powerlifting champion in the 205-pound class for the Natural Association of Strength Athletes, puts it this way:

$$\text{Understanding} + \text{energy} = \text{results}$$

"Many athletes waste a lot of time because they don't understand how the body works," says Elder. "You don't need a biochemistry degree, but you do have to appreciate what stimulates the body to grow. Yet, it's what you do with this information that really counts. Find the time to apply this knowledge in a disciplined way to your workouts and follow the formula consistently. Harness your energy so that it becomes a tool for achieving your goals. Without this controlled approach, much of your training energy will be wasted."

Discipline is necessary to make sure that your training program is geared to your body's ability to respond and recuperate. Instead of impulsively doing every exercise you can think of, you recognize your limits at a particular point of time. This way you don't feel compelled to keep up with the training volumes of your fellow athletes, which may or may not be optimal even for them. Muscle growth takes time, but the results are well worth the effort. Remembering this can give you the discipline to restrict the frequency and duration of your workouts. Your motto should be not too little, not too much. In the long run, this disciplined approach will bring you the greatest rewards.

39.

RESPECT THE EBB
AND FLOW OF LIFE

While training is an important part of your life, you probably have other commitments that seem to get in the way of your muscle-building goals. Don't be frustrated. Work, family, and friends add meaning to your life, too. By achieving a balance among these various activities, you will actually help your muscle growth. Don't try to force progress, either. When you get in sync with your life's patterns, you will feel more satisfaction and grow faster as well.

You've probably dreamed about a fantasy world in which nothing ever gets in the way of your training. It's a nice dream, but in the real world the chances of it happening are pretty slim. For most of us, we need to balance our desire to train with the other responsibilities in our lives. We often grudgingly accept this as an obligation, wishing that there were some other way. Yet, athletes with a balanced approach to life often out-perform athletes who let their lives get out of kilter. From this standpoint, balance is something that is essential to achieving your growth goals.

Balance exists when the various aspects of your life are in sync. Training does not totally dominate your life any more than work does. There is variety, with a career and social activities each adding to the total enjoyment in life. Even within your training regimen, routines are balanced between resistance training and aerobics, between indoor activities and outdoor ones. There is a balance between exercise and recuperation, and even between dietary strictness and that little splurge that gives you an emotional boost. This allows you to get the greatest satisfaction from your achievements, because you have the perspective to appreciate your accomplishments in a healthy way.

There are several ways to tell when your life is in balance. There are greater feelings of self-contentment and a healthier orientation toward life. Your outlook is more long-term, and you become more objective about the inevitable ups and downs that occur. Balance also leads to greater efficiency and productivity in work. You are able to focus 100 percent of your energies on the task at hand, without the daydreaming and poor mental focus that can come from an overdose of work or even training.

Progress does not occur in a straight, upward line. There are good days and bad days. Nothing can be more frustrating than not being able to lift as much as you did during your last workout. But don't get depressed. If the long-term direction of your lifting performance is upward, you have accomplished something that you can take great satisfaction in. However, if the trend is only level or negative, you may not be recuperating enough or your diet or stress level may be holding you back. Analyze the reasons for this and look for a balanced solution.

Work gives you money for the necessities of life and hopefully a few luxuries. At the same time, being a workaholic is bad for your physical and mental health. You need to strike a balance. If possible, modify your work habits and timetable in a way that will maximize growth. Spread out your work schedule so that it accommodates the demands of your training. Don't procrastinate until the last minute to finish your assignments. Plan ahead just as you'd do with your training, anticipating the demands that your boss and work associates will make on you. When things are slow at work, charge ahead with your training program. Then, when work demands must dominate, shift gears and temporarily switch your priorities. Always think long-term. These ebb and flow periods will balance out over time, allowing you to develop your physique and your career simultaneously. Don't get frustrated when you miss a training session because of your job. Everything will work out in the end. Meanwhile, focus on how good it will feel when you get to the gym again.

Remember to watch the foods you eat during busy work periods. Don't succumb to the temptation to eat junk food when you're in a hurry. Remember that your body grows during recuperation periods, not while you're at the gym. It only takes a few minutes to pack a lunch and some snacks with foods that are full of protein and low in fat. Healthy prepared meals are also available near most workplaces. Instead of seeking a release from the stress of your work by eating junk, remind yourself about the benefits of eating all that nutritious food.

The concept of balance also extends to friends and family. Spending time with these people enriches your life by opening your mind to new ideas and attitudes that will help you in life. While there is never enough time to do everything you want, a balance between your work, training and social/family commitments will make you a well-rounded person. Even better, it will give you the perspective and confidence you need to grow as an individual, both mentally and physically. A balanced approach to life will therefore help you to reach your full potential as an athlete.

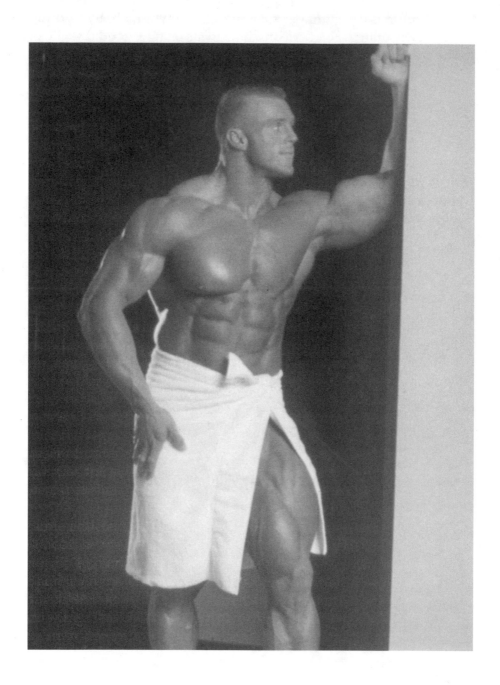

40.

RECUPERATE AND GROW

There is such a thing as too much training. You need to give your body the time it needs to recuperate from the physical demands of your workouts. Overtaxing your body's recuperative abilities will stop growth cold. Listen to the signals your body sends you, and never exercise a bodypart until it has not been sore for at least a day. Respect your body's ability to heal itself.

Athletes enjoy their training. Going to the gym is one of the highlights of their day, a time when they can make progress toward their goal of getting bigger and stronger. Taking time off is considered a negative. Our society constantly reinforces this mentality with its more-is-better philosophy. Athletes may feel that if some training is good, more must be better. Unfortunately, that's not how it works. If you don't give your body the time it needs to fully recuperate, your muscles will not grow. When it comes to building your body, there is such a thing as too much.

Only you can determine the frequency and duration of training that is right for you. No one system works for everyone because individual bodies vary. There are also individual differences in the stress levels produced by work and emotional relationships. This stress often prolongs the recuperation process by releasing catabolic hormones. Of course, it is essential to get the raw materials that your body needs for muscular growth. However, proper nutrition is not enough. You can eat all the protein you want and get plenty of vitamins and minerals, but without adequate recuperation your muscle development will be stuck in neutral.

"You need to respect your body's ability to heal," says exercise physiologist Karl List. "Step back every once in a while to gain perspective on your training. Your diet, work stress and amount of rest all impact the quality of your workouts. Things change, so maintain an open mind. Get plenty of rest and tailor your exercise program to your body's recuperation potential."

By and large, when you are at the gym you should train at peak intensity. Going through the motions with the same weight and the same number of repetitions you always do will not get you anywhere. Your body will just be repeating something it has done many times before. It's better to take a day or two off and fully recuperate so you can lift more weight than ever before when you return to the gym. This increased intensity will help to pack on more mass.

While muscle soreness is not a direct factor in muscular growth, it is an indication that you have trained the muscle hard enough to cause the adaptations needed for size gains. In this sense, some temporary soreness is good. However, if you're constantly sore, you're getting too much of a good thing. Soreness results from microscopic tears in the muscle fibers and other factors. This damage at the cellular level is repaired as the muscle grows. Yet, if you exercise so much that your body is always sore, you never give your muscles the time they need to recuperate and grow.

Never exercise a bodypart until it has *not* been sore for at least a day. If you find that applying this rule gets in the way of your current workout program, try stretching out your training schedule. Some athletes have changed from the traditional two- or three-day division of bodyparts to a four-day division of bodyparts. Others have added rest days between or during each bodypart rotation. Both of these variations lengthen the period between training sessions for a particular bodypart and increase the time available for recuperation.

Another option is to cut down on the number of sets for each bodypart. This way there is less stress on the muscle from each exercise session and less time needed for recovery. Remember that the muscle grows from peak intensity, not from an excessive volume of training. If you lift a few sets at your maximum weight and then find that the weights you can use keep dropping and dropping, you're better off stopping your bodypart workout right there. You're not going to grow from a few more sets at lighter weight. On the contrary, these extra sets will just increase the amount of recovery needed. Try experimenting with the number of sets to see how your muscles recuperate. You may find that they grow more with fewer sets.

A third option is to utilize what powerlifting coach Kurt Elder calls the "wave method." "Your body can't give 100 percent all of the time. Your muscles, joints and tendons need time to recuperate before your body can grow. Reduce the intensity and volume of your training periodically so you can form a solid foundation for future growth. It may seem like a step back, but in the final analysis you will accomplish your goals sooner than you would otherwise." This technique is also known as periodization.

Regardless of the method you choose, always keep in touch with your body. It will send you signals when it needs recuperation. Listen to them. Athletes often ignore these signals, figuring that they have to force the body to grow. Nothing could be further from the truth. By working with your body and giving it the recuperation it seeks, you will achieve the quickest muscle growth.

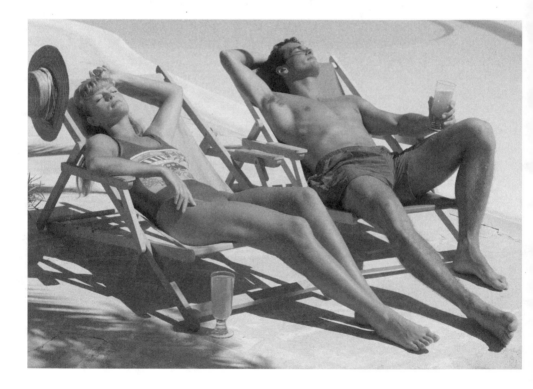

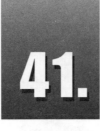

41.

GET ENOUGH SLEEP

Much of the body's recuperation process occurs during the sleeping hours. The greatest release of growth hormone also takes place at this time. You can't make up for lost sleep, so try to get seven to eight hours every night. If possible, go to sleep at the same time each day.

Sleep is a vital part of the recuperation process. The body requires sleep to perform at its best. Many of the benefits derived from sleep actually occur in the first few hours. It is during this period that most people fall into a deep sleep and the repair process operates at full speed. The greatest release of growth hormone also takes place during these initial hours of sleep.

Different people have different sleep requirements. Some people get along on as little as five or six hours, while others require at least eight. The reasons for this individual variation are still not known, although metabolism seems to be partly responsible. Weight training increases the amount of sleep required as the body works to fully recuperate before the next training session. If too much additional sleep is required, however, the body may well be signaling you that you are overtraining. This may result in sleeping through a radio alarm that normally would wake you up or other abnormalities. Overtraining can also reduce the quality of sleep by disturbing sleep patterns and even waking the athlete up during the night. If your muscles are so sore that you wake up every time you move in bed, this will also reduce the effectiveness of your sleeping hours.

As a general rule, you should sleep seven to eight hours each day. The body cannot store sleep, and it can't catch up on lost sleep either. Therefore, it is essential to get the sleep you need every night. You can't spend Saturday night out on the town and wake up at your usual time, figuring that you'll catch up on this sleep during the week. It doesn't work that way. The body also seems to perform at its best when sleep takes place at roughly the same time every day. This provides a continuity that the body thrives on. Factory workers on rotating shifts have often noticed that the quality of their sleep is affected by radical changes in the times of day they rest, even when the actual number of hours slept remains the same. You should try to minimize these shifts in sleep patterns. This will allow your body's muscle development system to operate at peak efficiency, ensuring you the maximum benefit from all of your hard work.

42.

BE PATIENT

Rome wasn't built in a day, and your body won't be either. We all wish we could snap our fingers and get huge, but it doesn't work that way. Muscle growth occurs in spurts, so don't get discouraged. Patience is a virtue. If your training program and diet are appropriate, you will eventually achieve the muscle mass you are looking for.

Athletes are impatient by nature. They tend to be action-oriented individuals who enjoy a fast-paced lifestyle. Words such as easygoing and laid-back are rarely used to describe men and women who take the time to build up their bodies. Waiting is for other people. Athletes know what they want, and they want it now.

Of course, this drive is often a positive virtue. Once you establish your muscle-building goals, you want to pursue them with total intensity. However, you need to remember that your body has its limits. The mind may be willing to constantly push the body to the edge, and for a while the body may be willing to go along. But inevitably the time comes when the body protests what it considers abuse. Your strength will stop increasing and may even decrease. If you continue in your ways, you could give yourself a cold or other illness, which will set back your training by several weeks, at best. You need to be patient. All good things come in time.

Be realistic about the amount of time it will take to reach your physique goals. Athletes sometimes set themselves up for disappointment by using unrealistic timetables for their muscle growth. When you first start training, you will experience relatively rapid increases in your strength and mass. This is due to the initial neuromuscular adaptations that occur when the body first "learns" how to work out. These rapid changes are very encouraging, but they can lead some athletes to expect equivalent gains over the long term. Unfortunately, the rate of growth decreases as time goes on. You need to resist the temptation to continually increase your volume of training in an attempt to keep your gains on track. Building the ideal physique takes time. If you pile on so much intensity that you wind up overtraining, it will take even more time.

Muscle growth occurs in spurts. For reasons that are still not totally understood, the body's adaptations to exercise do not have a direct relationship with the amount of effort expended. There are, of course, hormonal fluctuations that occur over time. Changes in your diet can also be a factor, as can variations in stress levels and other lifestyle considerations. Yet even taking these factors into account, you will likely experience periods when you seem to grow quickly and other times when your size gains appear to be minimal or nonexistent. Don't give up just yet. Exercise a bit of self-control and perseverance. Patiently continue with your current workout program for a while. It may not be the reason for your lack of growth.

If this situation continues for an extended period, you will need to change your training, diet or supplementation variables, and this book provides you with many different ways to enhance the effectiveness of your training. However, once again you need to be patient. Don't presume that a workout variation is useless when you don't see growth in the first week or even month. These things take time. Continue with your new training variable for three months before moving on to the next change. If you constantly alter your training, diet or supplementation variables, you will never be able to figure out what works for you and what doesn't. Persistence and tenacity will help you determine your ideal workout program.

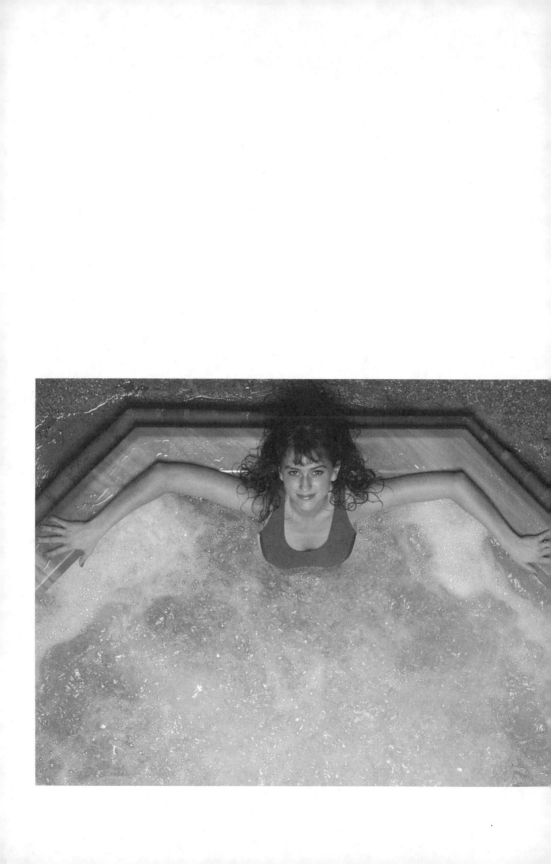

43.

KEEP YOUR STRESS LEVEL LOW

Stress can reduce your muscle growth or even stop it altogether. The body responds to stress by releasing the catabolic hormone cortisol. Stay on the anabolic path by keeping your stress level as low as possible. Exercise is one of many ways to decrease stress and anger. When you feel stressed, deal with it right away.

It was once felt that only viral and bacterial agents impacted the immune system. Now, scientists recognize that the mind influences its strength and functioning. Too much worrying can literally make you sick. Muscle growth, of course, requires a healthy immune system. When anabolic forces predominate in the body, growth is maximized. When stress rears its ugly head, however, the body responds by releasing the catabolic hormone cortisol. To keep your growth on track, you need to find ways to control your stress level.

Many athletes find it hard to relax. Things move at such a rapid pace nowadays that there never seems to be enough time to do all of the things you want to. Your only option is to learn to relax in the limited time you have available. There are many different relaxation techniques. Weight training can be an excellent way to reduce stress if you do it properly. If you feel stressed out from work, concentrate on your sets. Escape into the exercise. Let it become your total reality for a minute or two. If you are angry with your boss, use the anger to fuel your set. As you do each repetition, think "Take that, you #@%&!" Just be careful that you don't let your anger reduce the quality of your exercise, or you could injure yourself and really get frustrated! When you properly channel your emotions, you'll be surprised how quickly your stress and anger can evaporate. By the time you leave the gym, those negative feelings may be a distant memory.

Everyone feels stressed out from time to time. It's an unfortunate part of modern living. Yet, you can dramatically reduce your stress level by following a few simple guidelines. The first step is to get in touch with your own feelings. Keep a diary of the events that produce stress for you. Then analyze each of them to see how you could alter the situation or at least change the way you respond to it. If you get stressed out waiting in line at the bank, rearrange your schedule to go when the bank isn't busy. Or at least bring a magazine to pass the time while you work your way up the line. You'll be talking to the teller before you know it.

There are many more ways to reduce stress. You could enjoy a sunset for a few minutes. Counting to ten or breathing slowly may also work. There are more structured forms of relaxation therapy including yoga, tai chi, and several other disciplines from the East that can help you achieve a more relaxed approach to life. One of the better ways to get rid of stress is also the most enjoyable: Do something nice for yourself. This special thing doesn't have to be a world cruise, either. Little things are just as effective. Get a massage or sneak away to that secret hiding place that only you know about. Try a steam bath, sauna, or Jacuzzi. Sometimes even reminiscing about a pleasant experience in your past will reduce your stress.

Your attitude plays a big role in your stress level. Clearly, the way you approach life has a big impact on your experiences. Look on the bright side. If there are no parking spaces near your gym, don't blow your top. Park a block away and get to know the neighborhood better. Do some window-shopping, or chat with a friend you meet along the way. You could even get in a bit of warm-up by jogging or walking briskly to the gym door. It all works out in the end. When you approach life with a balanced, positive attitude, you reduce your stress level and do your body a world of good.

When you feel stress coming on, deal with it as soon as possible. Try one of these stress-reduction techniques or come up with another of your own. If you feel stress frequently, look for a way to reduce the life situations that produce these feelings. There may be another option you haven't explored yet. When you get a lemon, make lemonade. Seek out the proverbial silver lining. Focus on the ways that you can actually change your life. Things are rarely as hopeless as they appear at the time.

Never accept stress as part of your reality. Go out and change things. The positive feelings that result will put your mind back into an anabolic mode and invigorate your training sessions, producing renewed muscle growth.

44.

LIMIT ALCOHOL USE

Excessive alcohol consumption can reduce your muscle gains. Alcohol decreases the secretion of growth hormone while lengthening recovery time. It has even been shown to shrink the muscle fibers of alcoholics. If you frequently use alcohol, cutting back on your consumption will produce a more anabolic environment for muscle growth.

Athletes occasionally drink beer or wine to relax on weekends or after a hard day's work. Like many other people, they enjoy the temporary stress reduction and the "buzz" they get from a drink or two. Within reason, this practice appears to be harmless. There is no evidence that the sporadic consumption of alcohol produces a significant restriction on muscle growth. However, if you use alcohol daily or in large quantities on weekends, you may be holding back your size gains.

Alcohol (or ethanol, as it is known technically) has many different effects in the body. It is used medically as a sedative and to reduce fever and pain. This is why it appears in numerous medications for the common cold. The recreational use of alcohol, however, can make it harder to build muscle. Alcohol has been shown to increase recovery time from the stresses of exercise. It reduces the secretion of growth hormone from the pituitary gland as well. Both of these effects keep the body from building structural muscle proteins as quickly as would otherwise be possible.

A review study by Martin and Peters also noted a selective atrophy (or shrinkage) of the fast-twitch muscle fibers in alcoholics. These fibers are the ones that increase the most in size with weight training. While the moderate use of alcohol will not have such a negative effect, it seems clear that alcohol does not do your muscles any good. Your body may well be able to overcome the restraints that alcohol places on growth, but the energy it expends to do so might be put to better use. There is no free lunch. You need to ask yourself whether the benefit you get from alcohol is worth the cost.

Of course, the negative impact of alcohol is dose-related. A drink or two will not have a demonstrable effect on your muscle growth. On the other hand, ask anyone with a hangover how anabolic they feel and how strong they are that day. If you frequently drink alcohol, cutting back on your consumption will remove a restraining factor for your muscle development. Don't rationalize your beer drinking by thinking it's made from whole grains and contains protein. It is better to experience the "exercise high" from the endorphins released during exercise instead. You'll feel better and grow more as well.

45.

EASE INTO YOUR TRAINING AFTER AN ILLNESS

Athletes frequently resume their full-intensity workouts as soon as they get over a cold or other illness. Some even feel they can "sweat out" a virus. These practices strain your recovering immune system and can cause a relapse. It's better to ease into your training program. This will give your body a chance to fully recuperate and in the long run will stimulate more growth.

Athletes have a hard time dealing with illness. They feel that they are entitled to perpetual good health because of their physical activities at the gym. After all, compared to many people in the general population, athletes eat better and have a healthier lifestyle. In some people's minds, this should eliminate the chances of getting colds, sore throats and other viral and bacterial infections. However, this is clearly not the case. Many athletes have been known to overtrain, which reduces the strength of their immune systems and permits an infection or other illness to take hold. These afflictions can also impact men and women who do not overtrain, although it tends to happen less frequently.

When athletes do become sick, they often respond poorly. They fear that they will lose precious time in their efforts to gain size. This can even lead to depression and a sense of futility as they react to this negative twist of fate. Should these pessimistic thoughts enter your mind, cast them aside. Focus on the long term. Life is a roller-coaster ride, so don't lose perspective. Instead of dwelling on the inequities of life, try to determine why you got sick in the first place. Viruses and other "bugs" are in the air most of the time, so something must have temporarily lowered your immunity. If the answer relates to your diet, training program, stress level or environmental variables, make a commitment to change these factors in the future.

Athletes frequently try to do a full-intensity workout as soon as they feel slightly better. Some even return to the gym while they still have a fever, figuring that they can "sweat out" the responsible virus. These counterproductive practices have caused far too many relapses. Premature training reduces the body's resistance and can actually prolong the amount of time you feel under the weather. It's better to take a bit more time off to regain your strength. In the long run, you will recuperate more quickly and reach your previous strength levels more rapidly.

Once you are ready to return to the gym, ease into your training program. Think of your temporary setback as a form of periodization and cut back on the amount of weight you lift for a while. Start at approximately 60 percent of your previous lifts and do as many repetitions as you can without putting a great deal of stress on the muscle. Now is not the time to force out that very last rep! Although the thrill of being back in the gym may encourage you to train to the point of exhaustion, restrict your training volume to no more than six sets each for arms, shoulders, calves and abs and nine sets each for chest, back and legs. Your immune system is still weak, so work with your body. When you treat it right, it will treat you right.

During your second week back, increase your training intensity to 75 percent of your former lifts. Utilize the same routine you were using before your illness. For the next bodypart cycle increase the weights you use to 90 percent, then go to 100 percent of your previous limit. Now exceed your former limits and achieve new levels of strength and muscle mass. You're back on the track to muscle growth! Savor it and be thankful for your renewed good health. But remember the lessons you learned about your body's limits and respect them in the future. This will keep the time you lose to illness to a minimum.

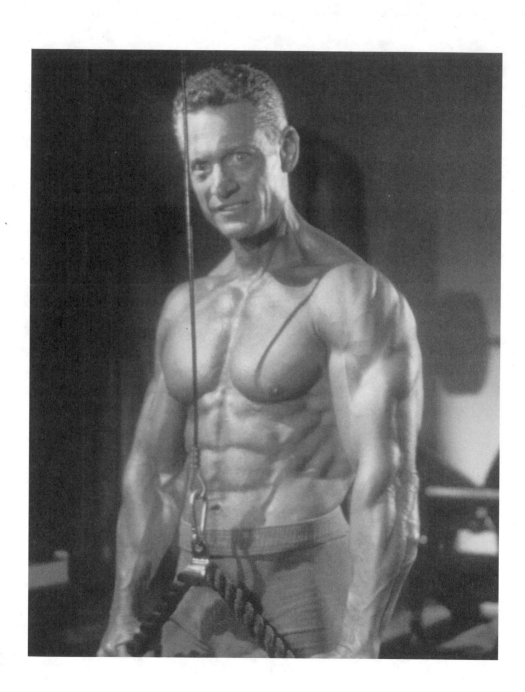

46.

LEARN FROM YOUR MISTAKES

One of life's certainties is that you will make mistakes. The important thing is to learn from them. Experiment with your workouts to determine the ideal program for you. Try different diet and supplementation regimens, too. Don't get depressed if you occasionally screw up. You need to explore alternatives in order to be on the cutting edge of growth.

Everyone makes mistakes. To err is human, as they say, but there's no use crying over spilt beer. The important thing is to learn from your mistakes, drawing conclusions from your past experiences that will enable you to never make the same mistake again. This is true for life in general, and it is certainly true when it comes to muscle growth. You have to listen to your body and respect the signals that it sends you.

In order to maximize your size gains you need to experiment with your training program. This experimentation will enable you to establish the proper frequency and volume of exercise for you. You have to use heavy weight judiciously. While you must push the limit in your workouts in order to stimulate growth, too much stimulation is counterproductive. Learn from your mistakes and alter your training accordingly. Isolate the factors that seem to work for you and incorporate them into your workouts. Observe the responses that your body makes to the stimuli you offer it, then retain the good and discard the bad. This process will be somewhat different for each athlete, so be prepared to individualize your training program. Don't be afraid to do something that's different, for only through trial and error can progress be made.

Some machines at the gym will work better for you than others. By necessity, machines are designed for a hypothetical average person. This is great provided that you match the dimensions of this person, but if you're taller or shorter the machine may not work as designed. It may even cause strain or injury, so you need to pick and choose among the available options. Diet is another area for experimentation. Metabolisms vary, so the amount of carbs you need to grow without gaining bodyfat will also vary. Through the learning process you will determine what works best for you.

You need to maintain a positive conviction that you will excel, not in spite of your mistakes but actually because of them. People who don't experiment and take chances will never learn as quickly as they might. They will never be on the cutting edge of sports or anything else for that matter. No risk, no reward. Be bold in your experiments, but remember to use your intellect, intuition and common sense. You can't make uncommon gains if you do the same thing that everyone else does. In order to grow mentally and physically you have to take charge of your destiny and be your own master. Make change your friend, but don't throw out the baby with the bath water. While you will sometimes screw up, as long as you don't get negative and short-circuit the process you will benefit from your individualized program. In time you will experience the full satisfaction and rewards of muscle growth.

47.

REMAIN
CONFIDENT

A confident attitude increases your mental and physical power. Instead of doubting your ability to excel, you push forward with strength and conviction. Confidence is different than arrogance. It is the recognition that you can set the limits for your achievement. Don't let the negative aspects of life get you down. Remain confident and you will grow faster.

Nobody is confident 100 percent of the time. We all know how it feels to be uncertain and apprehensive about how our training and lives are going. Yet, you have the power to direct your thoughts in an optimistic and productive direction.

You need to selectively interpret the world around you. Think of the proverbial glass as half full instead of half empty. By looking on the bright side you can develop the confidence that will let you achieve your mass-building goals. "Your body will do whatever your mind wants it to," says exercise physiologist Karl List. "You have to be willing to knock on the door of opportunity hard enough. Tune in to your desire for muscle growth and never let doubt enter your mind. If you think the door only opens so far, you'll never reach your destination. Confidence in your abilities will maximize your growth potential."

There is a big difference between confidence and arrogance. You have no doubt seen your share of cocky, arrogant people at the gym. Yet, arrogance (or attitude, as it's sometimes called) actually shows a lack of self-confidence. A truly confident individual does not need to impress people with endless bragging. Real confidence comes from within. It is self-contained and much more powerful. Arrogance will hold you back, but confidence will release a new level of mental and physical strength that you didn't even know you had.

Building confidence is easy provided that you make the effort. After all, no one is born confident. This personality trait is developed over the years, usually with encouragement from parents and peers. You can increase your confidence level in several ways. First, take pride in your past accomplishments. Even though you probably haven't gotten everything you've hoped for, you have still accomplished a great deal. Every athlete's life is full of successes. You need to focus on the positive things that have happened so far in your life.

Second, make a list of your new accomplishments each week. Perhaps you added another plate to your leg press or upped the weight on your dumbbell curls. Maybe you lost a pound of bodyfat for the fifth week in a row. It doesn't have to qualify for the history books to have meaning for you. Whatever it is, acknowledge it and savor the victory.

Third, set short-term goals and make them happen. While you need a long-term goal to maintain direction in your training, it's best to divide that goal into short-term, more readily attainable goals. This way you get ongoing positive feedback and the wonderfully confident feeling of goal achievement.

Fourth, remain confident in the face of failure. Being human, you will sometimes fail in what you set out to do, but remember that no one has a perfect record. Analyze your expectations to see whether they were realistic to start with. It may be that you have succeeded in most people's eyes, even if it doesn't feel that way to you. If your first plan doesn't work, confidently replace it with another. Failure most often stems from a lack of persistence.

Develop a new training strategy and stick with it. Confidently pursue your dream.

Finally, don't let other people's lack of confidence rob you of yours. There are a lot of negative people in the world, and they would like nothing better than to drag you down to their level. The decision is yours. If you want to excel as an athlete, you have to block out this negativity and remain true to yourself. In the end, you will achieve your goals if you remain confident in your abilities.

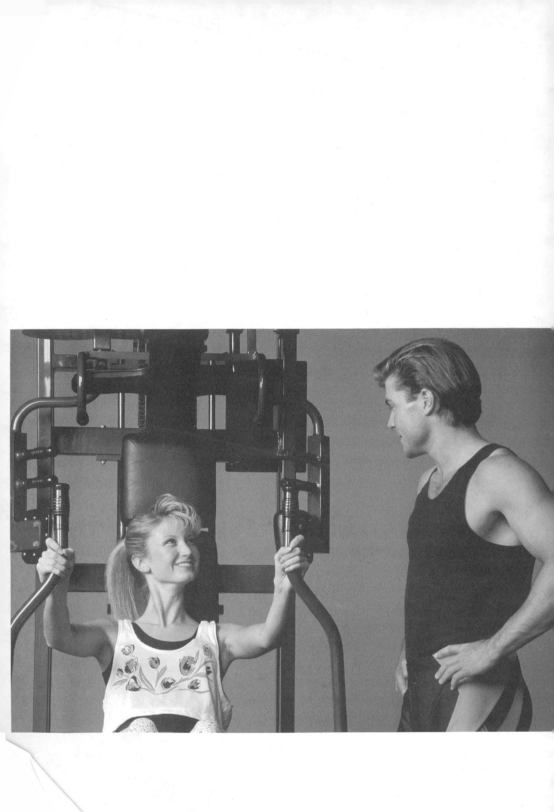

GET POSITIVE REINFORCEMENT

Building muscle is hard work, and the hardest part can be maintaining a constructive frame of mind. Maximize your motivation by getting positive reinforcement from the good people around you. Accept their compliments and use them to increase your training enthusiasm. Also, return the favor. Reinforcement works both ways.

In your quest to excel as an athlete, you need to pull out all of the stops when it comes to stimulating muscle growth. Your success is not preordained. Much as we would wish it otherwise, success takes time and effort. Yet, the rewards are great.

There will be times when your motivation is not all that it could be. You might be bored about life in general or because your muscle gains aren't coming as quickly as you would like. These negative thoughts can definitely impact your workouts. You can't have a superior training session when you feel as if you're getting the short end of the stick at the gym, at work or in your social life.

At times like this, you need to find reinforcement for your

long-term training goals. Don't just sit there and mope because things aren't perfect. This is the real world. Seek out reinforcement to help you on your path to muscle size and strength. This reinforcement can take many forms. Your friends could comment on your strength gains or how much you have grown lately. Your training partner could note how your new diet is taking hold, pointing out how your definition and vascularity are increasing with each passing day. Or a new person at the gym could catch your eye. When they smile back, you start up a conversation that leads to a friendship and (who knows) maybe more. The types of reinforcement are infinite and are dependent on your particular feelings and desires. Regardless of the specific action, however, reinforcement is very beneficial.

Positive reinforcement bolsters enthusiasm for your training. Getting a needed pat on the back will motivate you to hit the weights with renewed intensity. You will be able to drive past that pizzeria without even looking back, knowing that the short-term sacrifices you make will pay off big in the long run. Reinforcement will also boost your concentration. Instead of losing focus and dividing your available mental energy between negative thoughts and the workout at hand, you plunge into your workout with renewed stamina. Reinforcement provides confirmation of the progress you have made to date. You recognize that with drive and determination the future will bring more of the same, leading to more reinforcement from others. This will add still more vigor and vitality to your workouts, extending your capacity to grow.

Absorb the positive reinforcement you get while repelling the negative reinforcement around you. Spend your time with positive people like yourself who are willing to do what it takes to get the bodies they desire. Help them to achieve their goals, too. (Reinforcement works both ways!) You'll no doubt wind up with a much better physique and some solid friendships as well.

Always expect a positive outcome. It is preferable to expect success and occasionally be disappointed than to expect failure and be surprised when things work out well. Outcome expectancy is a valuable tool that is constantly at your disposal. Making excuses is easy. Muscle growth is hard work. So give yourself positive reinforcement every day and set yourself on a new path to size and strength.

49.

TAKE A VACATION FROM TRAINING SEVERAL TIMES A YEAR

Your body needs a break from the stresses of training every once in a while. Even with proper short-term recuperation, excessive amounts of exercise can be counterproductive over the long haul. During your time off, engage in other physical and social activities that will round out your life. This will reinvigorate your training once you return to the gym.

Athletes like going to the gym. Working out is not some dreary obligation that must be endured. For most athletes, training is one of the highlights of their day. So you may be hesitant to take time off from the gym. But anything in excess can be hazardous to your psychological or physical health in the long run. Also, anything in excess will eventually get boring as you tire of the routine. The way to ensure long-term training productivity is to maintain a healthy balance in your life's activities. This includes occasionally taking breaks from the rigors of your training routine.

"Training is very important," says powerlifting coach Kurt Elder, "but it shouldn't be the sum total of your life. We are carbon-based life forms who are only on this planet for a short time. You need to seek out other physical and social activities that will round out your life. While it may seem that these experiences can keep you from meeting your training objectives, they actually increase motivation and achievement over the long haul."

These vacations from training should occur at several times during the year. While the precise timing should be based on your own perceptions of need, don't rationalize that you really don't require a break. Looking back, you may realize how beneficial it actually was. This time-out from training does not have to take place while you are on your vacation from work. Many athletes have noticed that they get an excellent workout when they are in a new gym environment, particularly when they aren't mentally and physically drained from their jobs. So if you enjoy working out on your regular vacation, go ahead. Just be sure to set aside some time for active and passive relaxation when you are back home. Don't be concerned that these activities will keep you from achieving your long-term physique goals. On the contrary, they will reinvigorate your training by promoting a sense of balance in your life.

Some of the athletes with the greatest longevity in their sports have had outside interests. Bill Pearl, who competed for many years as a bodybuilder, has an antique car collection. John Grimek, Mr. America in 1940 and 1941, was a fan of the opera. Of course, you may not be into cars or soprano solos, but there is some interest you do have, even if you haven't developed it yet as a hobby or personal activity. Try using your vacation time to make it a more significant part of your life. You will find that it actually helps your training by giving you another outlet for your energies. This should allow you to focus more fully on your training during the times when it is your primary activity, since it will be a variation from the other aspects of your life.

When it comes to your physical activities, spend this vacation time doing a variety of sports or interests. For example, you might occasionally try some rock climbing, mountain biking or even canoeing or river rafting. Some people might say that these "diversions" hold back the athlete from his or her training goals, but this balance in physical activities actually helps. Because there is more diversity in life, there will be a lot more mental stimulation. This will increase your level of achievement on the lifting platform, playing field or posing dais.

50.

CONTROL YOUR EGO

Ego is a double-edged sword. It can give you confidence and motivation, but it can also hold back your training progress. Don't go for the heaviest weight or an excessively long workout just because your ego wants a temporary boost. Your ultimate objective should be long-term ego gratification.

Ego can be a blessing or a curse. While a healthy amount of ego gives you inspiration and self-assurance, too much can actually hold you back. Proper channeling of the ego enhances your competitive spirit, but excessive ego can lead you to do things that are self-destructive. This can result in the selection of training techniques that reduce or even eliminate your strength and size gains.

The desire to lift the heaviest weight is strong. When you lift a heavy weight, you get an immediate ego boost. You feel so strong that you could take on the world. Yet, while you need to increase your weight loads over time to produce muscle growth, the ego's desire to jump to the largest dumbbell or the heaviest weight stack needs to be resisted. The fastest route to long-term gains is actually by making slower progressions in your weight levels over time. Big jumps in weight can rarely be sustained, and your ego will be bruised when you inevitably drop back. It's better to gently massage your ego with smaller yet continual weight gains than to set up your ego for a fall.

Don't be influenced by the "accepted truths" that you hear at the gym. You need to make your own personal decisions based on your body's ability to recuperate and grow. You shouldn't do something just because you see other people doing it. Those athletes may be responding to their own ego requirements without any thought of the implications of their actions.

Keep your form as perfect as possible, even if it means that you have to lower the amount of weight you lift to do so. The path to muscular greatness does not lie in the sloppy execution of an exercise movement. Weight levels that are too heavy invite injury, and you can't grow while you're out of action with a sprain or muscle tear. Also, restrict the volume of your training session even when your ego wants to set a new record for time spent in the gym. Your ego may be flying sky-high, but that is still no excuse to punish your muscle fibers with excessive numbers of sets. The athlete who avoids overtraining will be the one who achieves the quickest size increases.

Your ultimate objective should be long-term ego gratification, not counterproductive short-term fluffs. When you hit a plateau in your lifts, back off a bit to regroup. In the long run your muscles will welcome the respite and will reward you with solid gains. Once you learn to control your ego, you can use it as a positive force in your training program. So work with your ego and respect its power. It can be a valuable ally for growth.

CONCLUSION

This book has shown you how to design a muscle-building program that will let you develop your body to its maximum potential. You have seen the many ways in which your training regimen can be structured to increase muscular strength and size. You have learned the roles of diet and supplementation in providing the nutrients needed for muscle growth as well as the importance of lifestyle. You have also discovered how these variables interact in a synergistic way to produce the quickest gains.

The one remaining variable is you. Focus your physical and mental resources on the fulfillment of your muscular goals. Release all of your energies at the conscious and unconscious levels. Train with total intensity following a precise program that restricts the volume of training to your body's ability to recuperate and grow. Believe in the power of reinforcement and the inevitability of your physical improvement. Create forward motion by the strength of your will. Don't take the easy way out, because you will never get huge that way.

You now know how to build the physique you have dreamed about. The rest is up to you. Make your dream a reality!

Glossary

Anabolic. A metabolic process that results in a buildup of tissue or chemical compounds in the body.

Anoxia. A deficiency or complete cut-off of oxygen to specific tissues.

Catabolic. A metabolic process that causes the breakdown of tissue or chemical compounds in the body.

Compound set. Two exercises for the same bodypart that are performed without a rest in between.

Concentric movement. The phase of a repetition during which the muscle fiber is shortening. (Example: raising the weight during a biceps curl.)

Eccentric movement. The phase of a repetition during which the muscle fiber is lengthening. (Example: lowering the weight during a biceps curl.)

Isometric exercise. Any exercise where the person pushes against an immovable object.

Repetition. A single contraction of a muscle during a set, including the eccentric and concentric movements.

Set. One grouping of repetitions performed without a break

Super set. A set performed for a muscle on one side of a joint (agonist) followed immediately by a set for the muscle on the other side of this joint (antagonist). (Example: one set for biceps followed by one set for triceps, without rest in between.)

Index